DIABETIC

HEALTHY & DELICIOUS RECIPES

Publications International, Ltd.

Some of the products listed in this publication may be in limited distribution.

Pictured on the front cover *(clockwise from top left):* Greek Chicken Burgers with Cucumber Yogurt Sauce *(page 180)*, Chicken, Hummus and Vegetable Wraps *(page 49)*, and Broccoli Slaw with Chicken and Honey-Lime Dressing *(page 132)*.

Pictured on the back cover *(clockwise from top left):* Breakfast Quinoa *(page 5)*, Speedy Pineapple-Lime Sorbet *(page 263)*, and Mandarin Chicken Salad *(page 142)*.

ISBN: 978-1-68022-893-9

Library of Congress Control Number: 2017930974

Manufactured in China.

8 7 6 5 4 3 2 1

Nutritional Analysis: Every effort has been made to check the accuracy of the nutritional information that appears with each recipe. However, because numerous variables account for a wide range of values for certain foods, nutritive analyses in this book should be considered approximate. Different results may be obtained by using different nutrient databases and different brand-name products.

Microwave Cooking: Microwave ovens vary in wattage. Use the cooking times as guidelines and check for doneness before adding more time.

Note: This book is for informational purposes and is not intended to provide medical advice. Neither Publications International, Ltd., nor the authors, editors or publisher takes responsibility for any possible consequences from any treatment, procedure, exercise, dietary modification, action, or applications of medication or preparation by any person reading or following the information in this cookbook. The publication of this book does not constitute the practice of medicine, and this cookbook does not replace your physician, pharmacist or health-care specialist. **Before undertaking any course of treatment or nutritional plan, the authors, editors and publisher advise the reader to check with a physician or other health-care provider.**

Not all recipes in this cookbook are appropriate for all people with diabetes. Health-care providers, registered dietitians and certified diabetes educators can help design specific meal plans tailored to individual needs.

WARNING: Food preparation, baking and cooking involve inherent dangers: misuse of electric products, sharp electric tools, boiling water, hot stoves, allergic reactions, foodborne illnesses and the like, pose numerous potential risks. Publications International, Ltd. (PIL) assumes no responsibility or liability for any damages you may experience as a result of following recipes, instructions, tips or advice in this publication.

While we hope this publication helps you find new ways to eat delicious foods, you may not always achieve the results desired due to variations in ingredients, cooking temperatures, typos, errors, omissions, or individual cooking abilities.

CONTENTS

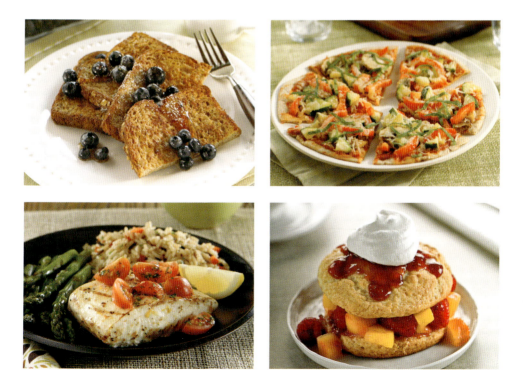

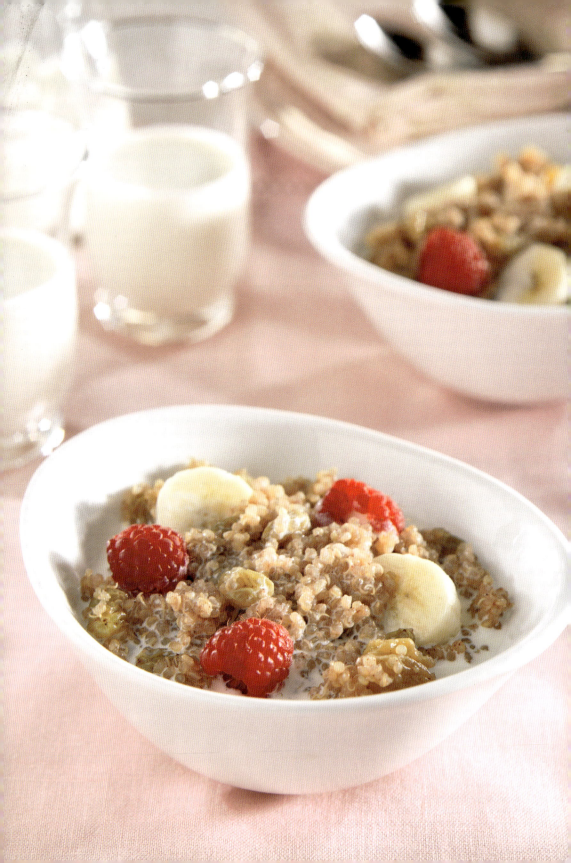

BREAKFAST & BRUNCHES

BREAKFAST QUINOA

Makes 2 servings

- ½ cup uncooked quinoa
- 1 cup water
- 1 tablespoon packed brown sugar
- 2 teaspoons maple syrup
- ½ teaspoon ground cinnamon
- ¼ cup golden raisins (optional)

  Milk (optional)

  Fresh raspberries and banana slices

1 Place quinoa in fine-mesh strainer; rinse well under cold running water. Transfer to small saucepan.

2 Stir in water, brown sugar, maple syrup and cinnamon; bring to a boil over high heat. Reduce heat to low; cover and simmer 10 to 15 minutes or until quinoa is tender and water is absorbed. Add raisins, if desired, during last 5 minutes of cooking. Serve with milk, if desired; top with raspberries and bananas.

Nutrition Information (per serving)

Calories 233, **Total Fat** 3g, **Saturated Fat** 1g, **Cholesterol** 0mg, **Sodium** 9mg, **Carbohydrates** 47g, **Dietary Fiber** 4g, **Protein** 6g

Dietary Exchanges: 2 Bread/Starch • 1 Fruit • ½ Fat

WHOLE WHEAT BLUEBERRY PANCAKES

Makes 4 servings (3 pancakes and about 2 tablespoons syrup per serving)

½ cup whole wheat pastry flour
½ cup all-purpose flour
1 teaspoon baking powder
½ teaspoon baking soda
⅛ teaspoon salt
1 cup low-fat (1%) buttermilk
1 large egg white, lightly beaten
1 tablespoon canola oil
1½ cups fresh blueberries, divided
½ cup sugar-free maple syrup

1 In medium bowl, combine both flours, baking powder, baking soda and salt. Stir in buttermilk, egg white and oil; mix just until dry ingredients are moistened. Stir in 1 cup blueberries.

2 Heat large nonstick skillet coated with nonstick cooking spray over medium heat. Drop batter by scant ¼ cupfuls into hot skillet. Cook 2 to 3 minutes or until bottoms are golden brown. Turn; cook 1 to 2 minutes longer or until bottoms are golden brown. Transfer to serving plates and keep warm in a 200°F oven while making remaining pancakes.

3 Combine remaining ½ cup blueberries and syrup in microwave-safe bowl; microwave on HIGH 20 to 30 seconds or until warm. Spoon over pancakes.

NOTE: Choose firm, plump blueberries with a silvery bloom. Avoid shriveled berries or berries with a green or red tint (an indication of an under-ripe berry). If the berries are packed in a clear plastic container, turn the container over and check for moldy or crushed berries.

Nutrition Information (per serving)

Calories 212, **Total Fat** 5g, **Saturated Fat** 1g, **Cholesterol** 2mg, **Sodium** 489mg, **Carbohydrates** 40g, **Dietary Fiber** 4g, **Protein** 7g

Dietary Exchanges: 1½ Bread/Starch • 1 Fruit • 1 Fat

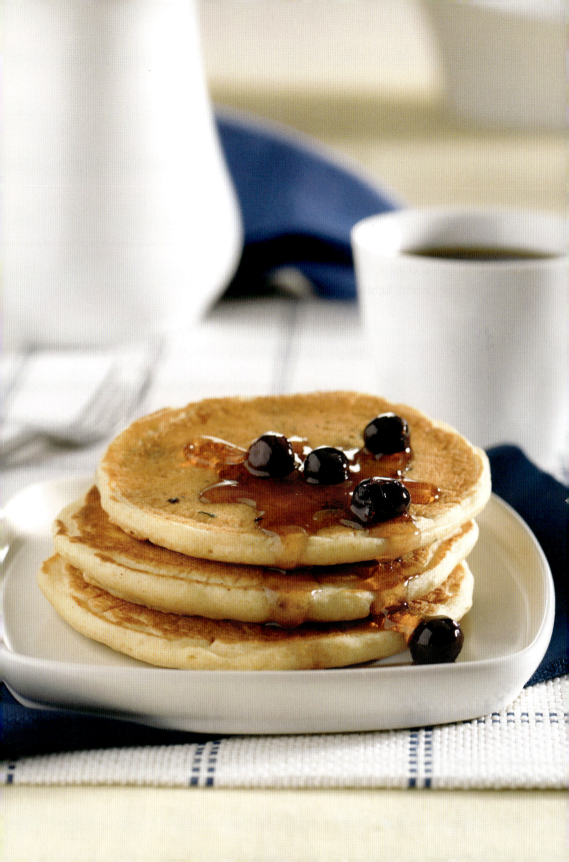

GERMAN APPLE PANCAKE

Makes 6 servings

1 tablespoon butter

1 large *or* 2 small apples, peeled and thinly sliced (about 1½ cups)

1 tablespoon packed brown sugar

1½ teaspoons ground cinnamon, divided

2 eggs

2 egg whites

1 tablespoon granulated sugar

1 teaspoon vanilla

¼ teaspoon salt

½ cup all-purpose flour

½ cup milk

Maple syrup (optional)

1 Preheat oven to 425°F.

2 Melt butter in medium cast iron or ovenproof skillet* over medium heat. Add apples, brown sugar and ½ teaspoon cinnamon; cook and stir 5 minutes or until apples just begin to soften. Remove from heat. Arrange apple slices in single layer in skillet.

3 Whisk eggs, egg whites, granulated sugar, remaining 1 teaspoon cinnamon, vanilla and salt in medium bowl until well blended. Stir in flour and milk until smooth and well blended. Pour evenly over apples.

4 Bake 20 to 25 minutes or until puffed and golden brown. Serve with syrup, if desired.

To make skillet ovenproof, wrap handle in foil.

NOTE: Pancake will fall slightly after being removed from the oven.

Nutrition Information (per serving)

Calories 120, **Total Fat** 2.5g, **Saturated Fat** 0.5g, **Cholesterol** 75mg, **Sodium** 160mg, **Carbohydrates** 18g, **Dietary Fiber** 1g, **Protein** 5g

Dietary Exchanges: 1 Bread/Starch • ½ **Fat**

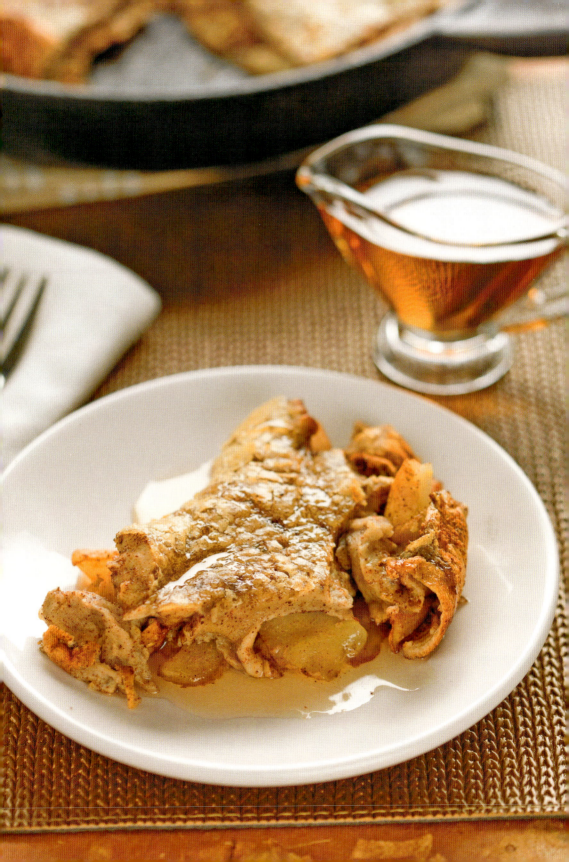

COTTAGE CHEESE BREAKFAST PARFAITS

Makes 4 servings

½ cup ½-inch diced cantaloupe cubes

½ cup ½-inch diced honeydew cubes

1 cup halved green or red seedless grapes

1 cup sliced fresh strawberries

1 container (16 ounces) low-fat (1%) cottage cheese

¼ cup toasted sliced almonds

Ground nutmeg (optional)

1 Combine cantaloupe, honeydew, grapes and strawberries in medium bowl.

2 Layer one third of cottage cheese in four short wide drinking glasses or wide wine glasses; top with half of fruit and half of almonds. Repeat layering with one third of cottage cheese, remaining fruit, remaining cottage cheese and remaining almonds. Sprinkle with nutmeg, if desired.

NOTE: This recipe is best if served immediately. Making the parfaits too far in advanced will cause the melon to weep into the cottage cheese.

Nutrition Information (per serving)

Calories 167, **Total Fat** 4g, **Saturated Fat** 1g, **Cholesterol** 5mg, **Sodium** 468mg, **Carbohydrates** 17g, **Dietary Fiber** 2g, **Protein** 16g

Dietary Exchanges: 2 Meat • 1 Fruit

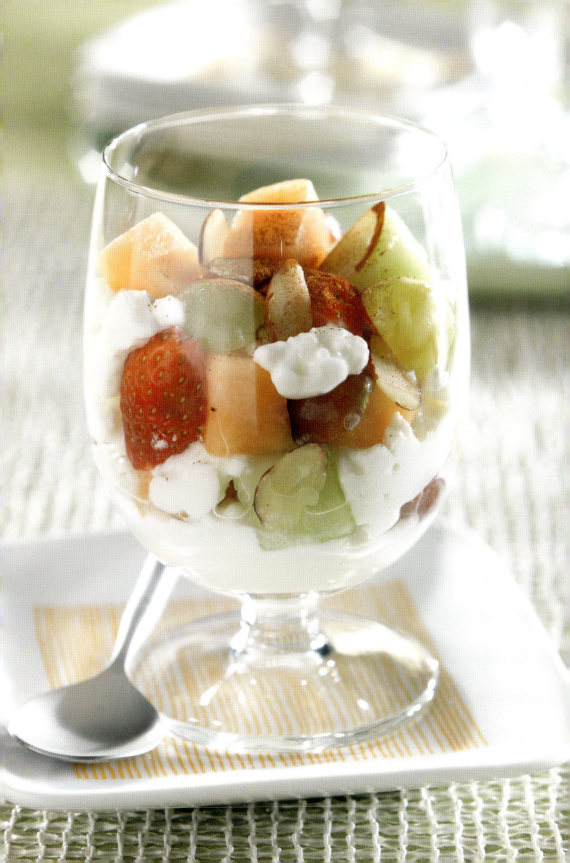

OVERNIGHT CHEESY VEGETABLE STRATA

Makes 10 servings

5 cups whole grain bread cubes (about 10 slices bread)

2 cups cooked broccoli, coarsely chopped

1 cup cooked mushrooms, chopped

½ cup sliced green onions

1¼ cups (5 ounces) shredded Swiss cheese, divided

2 cups cholesterol-free egg substitute

2 cups fat-free (skim) milk

1 tablespoon Dijon mustard

½ teaspoon black pepper

¼ teaspoon salt

1 Layer bread, broccoli, mushrooms and green onions in greased 13×9 baking dish. Sprinkle ¾ cup cheese evenly over vegetables.

2 Whisk egg substitute, milk, mustard, pepper and salt in medium bowl. Pour over strata. Refrigerate, covered, overnight.

3 Preheat oven to 350°F. Bake, uncovered, 30 minutes.

4 Sprinkle remaining ½ cup cheese evenly over top. Bake 10 to 12 minutes or until knife inserted into center comes out clean. Let stand 10 minutes before cutting and serving.

Nutrition Information (per serving)

Calories 180, **Total Fat** 5g, **Saturated Fat** 2.5g, **Cholesterol** 15mg, **Sodium** 370mg, **Carbohydrates** 19g, **Dietary Fiber** 1g, **Protein** 13g

Dietary Exchanges: 1 Bread/Starch • 1 Meat • ½ Vegetable • ½ Fat

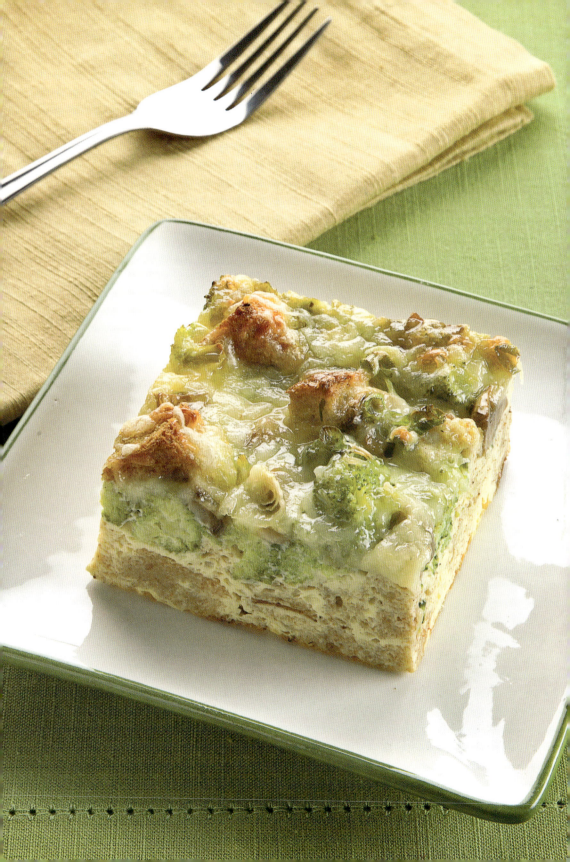

STRAWBERRY CINNAMON FRENCH TOAST

Makes 4 servings

1   **egg**

¼   **cup fat-free (skim) milk**

½   **teaspoon vanilla**

4   **(1-inch-thick) diagonally-cut slices French bread (about 1 ounce each)**

2   **teaspoons reduced-fat margarine, softened**

2   **packets sucralose-based sugar substitute***

¼   **teaspoon ground cinnamon**

1   **cup sliced fresh strawberries**

*This recipe was tested with sucralose-based sugar substitute.

1 Preheat oven to 450°F. Spray baking sheet with nonstick cooking spray.

2 Beat egg, milk and vanilla in shallow dish or pie plate. Lightly dip bread slices in egg mixture, coating completely. Place on prepared baking sheet.

3 Bake 15 minutes or until golden brown, turning halfway through baking time.

4 Meanwhile, combine margarine, sugar substitute and cinnamon in small bowl; stir until well blended. Spread mixture evenly over French toast; top with strawberries.

Nutrition Information (per serving)

Calories 125, **Total Fat** 3g, **Saturated Fat** 1g, **Cholesterol** 53mg, **Sodium** 220mg, **Carbohydrates** 19g, **Dietary Fiber** 2g, **Protein** 5g

Dietary Exchanges: 1 Bread/Starch • ½ Fat

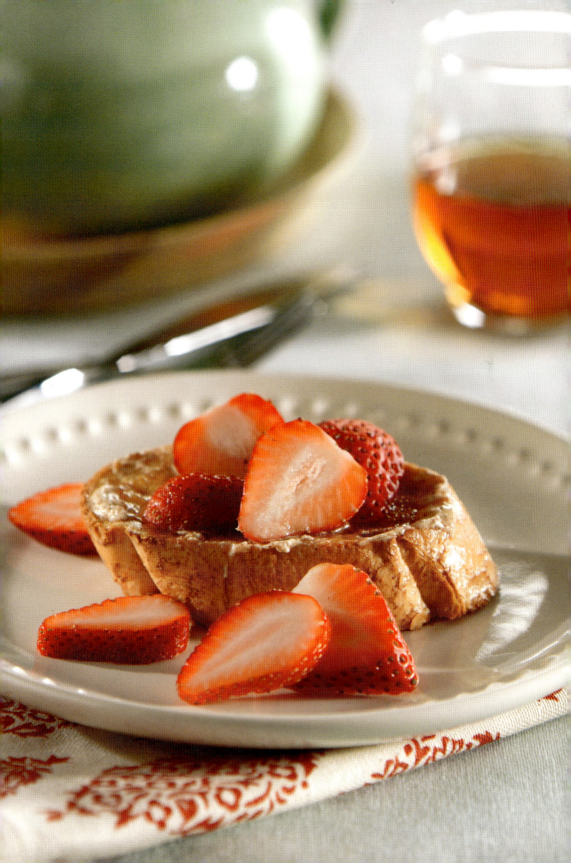

HAM AND VEGETABLE OMELET

Makes 4 servings

2 ounces (about ½ cup) diced 95% fat-free ham

1 small onion, diced

½ medium green bell pepper, diced

½ medium red bell pepper, diced

2 cloves garlic, minced

1½ cups cholesterol-free egg substitute

⅛ teaspoon black pepper

½ cup (2 ounces) shredded reduced-fat Colby cheese, divided

1 medium tomato, chopped

Hot pepper sauce (optional)

1 Spray 12-inch nonstick skillet with nonstick cooking spray; heat over medium-high heat. Add ham, onion, bell peppers and garlic; cook and stir 5 minutes or until vegetables are crisp-tender. Transfer mixture to large bowl.

2 Wipe out skillet with paper towels; spray with cooking spray. Heat over medium-high heat. Pour egg substitute into skillet; sprinkle with black pepper. Cook 2 minutes or until bottom is set, lifting edge of egg with spatula to allow uncooked portion to flow underneath. Reduce heat to medium-low; cover and cook 4 minutes or until top is set.

3 Gently slide omelet onto large serving plate; spoon ham mixture down center. Sprinkle with ¼ cup cheese. Carefully fold two sides of omelet over ham mixture; sprinkle with remaining ¼ cup cheese and tomato. Cut into four wedges; serve immediately with hot pepper sauce, if desired.

Nutrition Information (per serving)

Calories 126, **Total Fat** 4g, **Saturated Fat** 2g, **Cholesterol** 17mg, **Sodium** 443mg, **Carbohydrates** 8g, **Dietary Fiber** 1g, **Protein** 16g

Dietary Exchanges: 2 Meat • 1 Vegetable

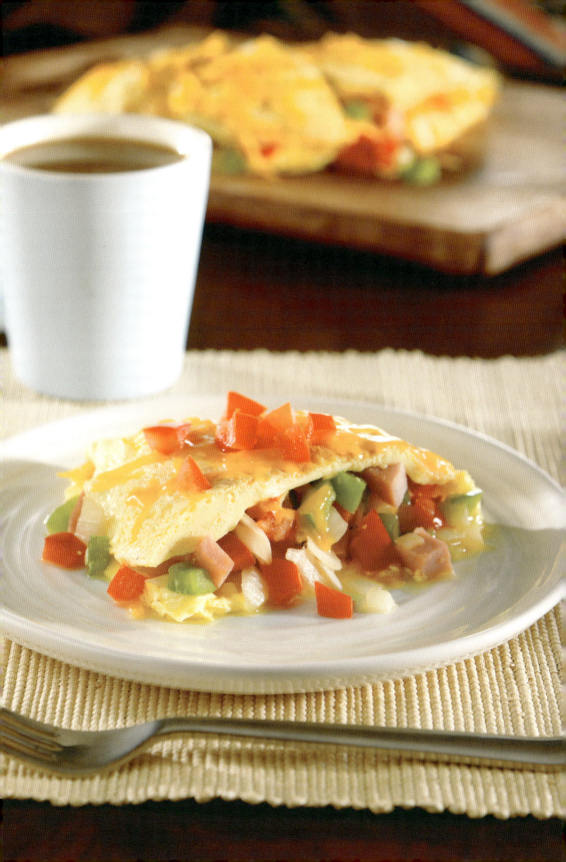

SKINNY SMOKED SALMON BAGELS

Makes 4 servings (1 bagel slice per serving)

2 whole wheat bagel thins*
   (4 bagel slices total)

2 ounces low-fat or whipped
   cream cheese

1 teaspoon dried dill weed

½ teaspoon Dijon mustard

1 ounce finely chopped red onion

2 ounces very thinly sliced
   smoked salmon, cut in thin
   strips or 2 ounces 96% extra-
   lean diced ham

*You may substitute with 2 sandwich thins or
scoop out the inside of 2 regular whole wheat
bagels.*

Lightly toast bagel slices. Meanwhile, whisk together cream cheese, dill and mustard in small bowl. Spread equal amounts of cream cheese mixture on each bagel slice, sprinkle evenly with onions and top with salmon or ham.

Nutrition Information (per serving)

Calories 116, **Total Fat** 5g, **Saturated Fat** 2g, **Cholesterol** 17mg, **Sodium** 454mg, **Carbohydrates** 14g, **Dietary Fiber** 3g, **Protein** 6g

Dietary Exchanges: 1 Bread/Starch • 1 Fat

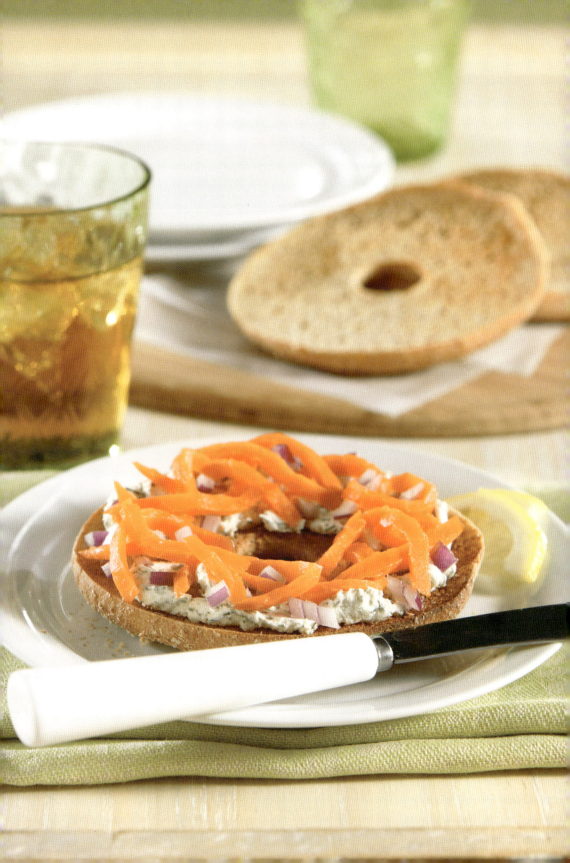

GREEN PEPPER SAUSAGE GRITS

Makes 4 servings (1 cup per serving)

2¼ cups water, divided

½ cup quick-cooking grits

¼ teaspoon salt, divided

6 ounces fully cooked turkey breakfast sausage links

2 teaspoons extra virgin olive oil

1 cup diced green bell pepper

1 cup grape tomatoes, quartered

2 cloves garlic, minced

¼ cup finely chopped green onions (green and white parts)

⅛ teaspoon ground red pepper

2 tablespoons chopped fresh parsley

1 Bring 2 cups water to a boil in medium saucepan over high heat. Gradually stir in grits; reduce heat. Cover and simmer 6 minutes or until thickened, stirring occasionally. Stir in ⅛ teaspoon salt. Set aside.

2 Meanwhile, spray large skillet with nonstick cooking spray; heat over medium-high heat. Add sausage; cook until browned, stirring to break up meat. Remove to plate.

3 Heat oil in same skillet over medium-high heat. Add bell pepper; cook and stir 3 minutes. Add tomatoes and garlic; cook 3 minutes or until softened. Stir in remaining ¼ cup water until well blended. Remove from heat.

4 Stir sausage and any accumulated juices, green onions, ground red pepper and remaining ⅛ teaspoon salt into skillet.

5 Divide grits among four serving plates. Top with sausage mixture and parsley.

Nutrition Information (per serving)

Calories 210, **Total Fat** 10g, **Saturated Fat** 3g, **Cholesterol** 26mg, **Sodium** 545mg, **Carbohydrates** 21g, **Dietary Fiber** 2g, **Protein** 9g

Dietary Exchanges: 1 Bread/Starch • 1 Meat • 1 Vegetable • ½ Fat

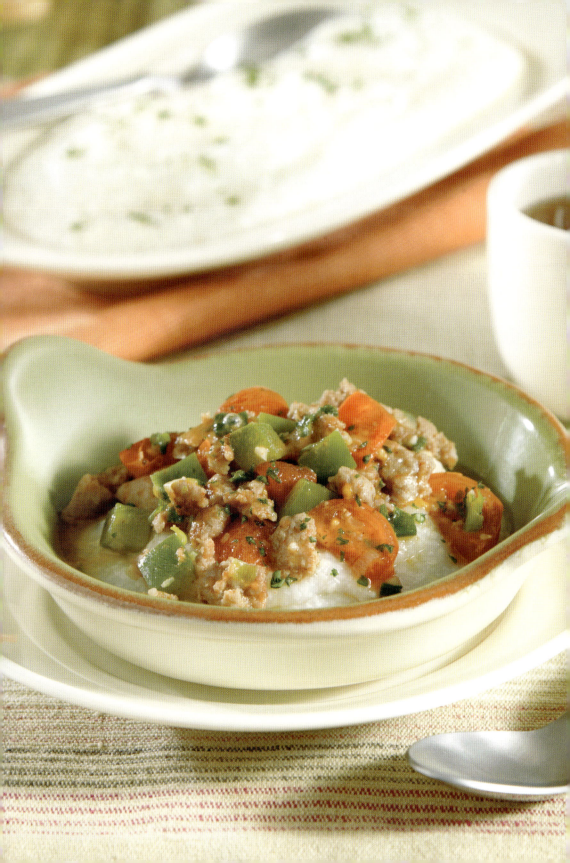

SPINACH, PEPPER AND OLIVE OMELET

Makes 4 servings (½ omelet per serving)

1 cup diced red bell pepper

½ teaspoon dried rosemary

⅛ teaspoon red pepper flakes

2 cups loosely packed baby spinach (2 ounces total), coarsely chopped

16 stuffed green olives, such as manzanilla, sliced

2 tablespoons chopped fresh basil

2 cups cholesterol-free egg substitute

3 tablespoons fat-free (skim) milk

2 ounces crumbled goat cheese or reduced-fat feta cheese, divided

1 Heat medium skillet coated with nonstick cooking spray over medium-high heat. Add bell pepper, rosemary and red pepper flakes; cook 4 minutes or until soft, stirring frequently. Remove from heat, stir in spinach, olives and basil; toss gently. Place in medium bowl, cover to allow spinach to wilt slightly and flavors to blend while preparing omelets.

2 Combine egg substitute and milk in another medium bowl; whisk until well blended. Wipe skillet clean with damp paper towel. Coat skillet with cooking spray and place over medium heat. Pour half of egg mixture into skillet. Cook 3 to 5 minutes, as eggs begin to set, gently lift edge of omelet with spatula and tilt skillet so uncooked portion flows underneath.

3 When egg mixture is set, spoon half of spinach mixture over half of omelet. Top with half of cheese. Loosen omelet with spatula and fold in half. Slide omelet onto serving plate and cover with foil to keep warm. Repeat with remaining ingredients.

Nutrition Information (per serving)

Calories 152, **Total Fat** 7g, **Saturated Fat** 3g, **Cholesterol** 11mg, **Sodium** 536mg, **Carbohydrates** 7g, **Dietary Fiber** 2g, **Protein** 16g

Dietary Exchanges: 2 Meat • 1 Vegetable

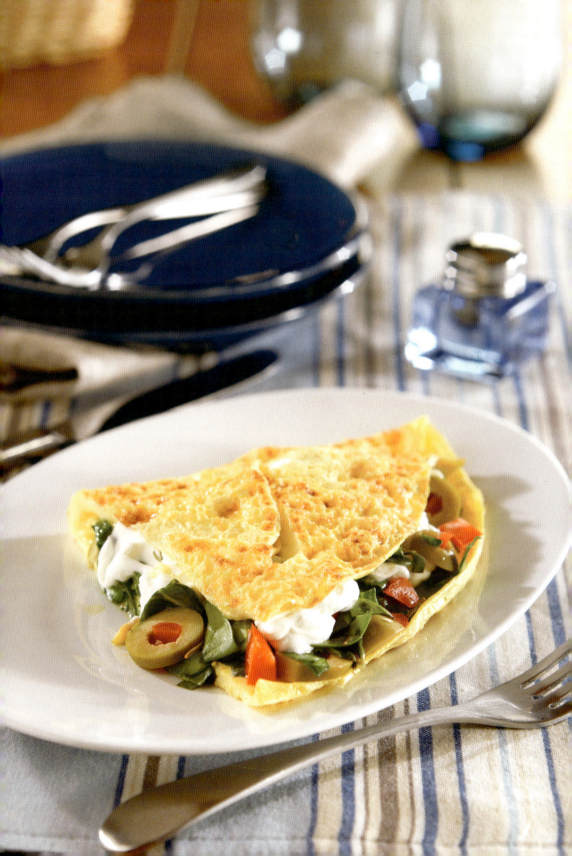

BREAKFAST COMFORT IN A CUP

Makes 4 servings (1 cup per serving)

4 teaspoons trans-fat-free margarine

4 slices reduced-calorie whole wheat bread, toasted

3 ounces 96% fat-free diced ham

1 cup cholesterol-free egg substitute

¼ cup (1 ounce) reduced-fat sharp Cheddar cheese, grated

¼ teaspoon black pepper

⅛ teaspoon salt (optional)

1 Spread 1 teaspoon margarine on each bread slice and cut into ½-inch cubes.

2 Meanwhile, heat large skillet coated with nonstick cooking spray over medium heat. Add ham and cook 3 minutes or until beginning to lightly brown, stirring occasionally. Add egg substitute, tilt skillet to coat bottom and stir occasionally until almost set. Fold in toast cubes, cheese, pepper and salt, if desired.

3 Spoon equal amounts in each of four cups, bowls or travel mugs.

NOTE: This low-carb breakfast will keep you going throughout the morning. You can even eat it on-the-go!

TIP: For a variation, you may substitute diced ham with turkey breakfast sausage links.

Nutrition Information (per serving)

Calories 130, **Total Fat** 4g, **Saturated Fat** 2g, **Cholesterol** 16mg, **Sodium** 550mg, **Carbohydrates** 12g, **Dietary Fiber** 3g, **Protein** 13g

Dietary Exchanges: ½ Bread/Starch • 2 Meat

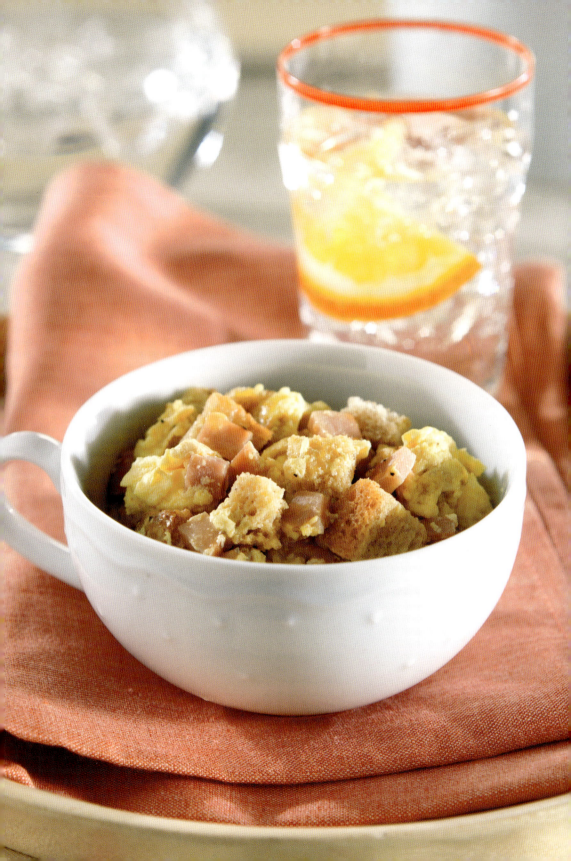

PB BANANA MUFFINS

Makes 18 muffins

- ¾ cup all-purpose flour
- ¾ cup whole wheat flour
- 1 teaspoon baking soda
- ½ teaspoon salt
- ¾ cup reduced-fat creamy peanut butter
- 2 ripe bananas, mashed (about 1 cup)
- ½ cup packed brown sugar
- ½ cup plain nonfat yogurt
- 1 egg
- ¼ cup honey
- ¼ cup vegetable oil
- 1 teaspoon vanilla

1 Preheat oven to 375°F. Line 18 standard (2½-inch) muffin cups with paper baking cups or spray with nonstick cooking spray.

2 Combine all-purpose flour, whole wheat flour, baking soda and salt in medium bowl; mix well. Beat peanut butter, bananas, brown sugar, yogurt, egg, honey, oil and vanilla in large bowl with electric mixer at medium speed until smooth and well blended. Add flour mixture; beat on low speed just until combined. Spoon batter evenly into prepared muffin cups.

3 Bake 15 to 18 minutes or until toothpick inserted into centers comes out clean. Cool in pans 5 minutes. Remove to wire racks; cool completely.

Nutrition Information (per serving)

Calories 184, **Total Fat** 8g, **Saturated Fat** 1g, **Cholesterol** 10mg, **Sodium** 223mg, **Carbohydrates** 25g, **Dietary Fiber** 2g, **Protein** 4g

Dietary Exchanges: 1½ **Bread/Starch** • 1½ **Fat**

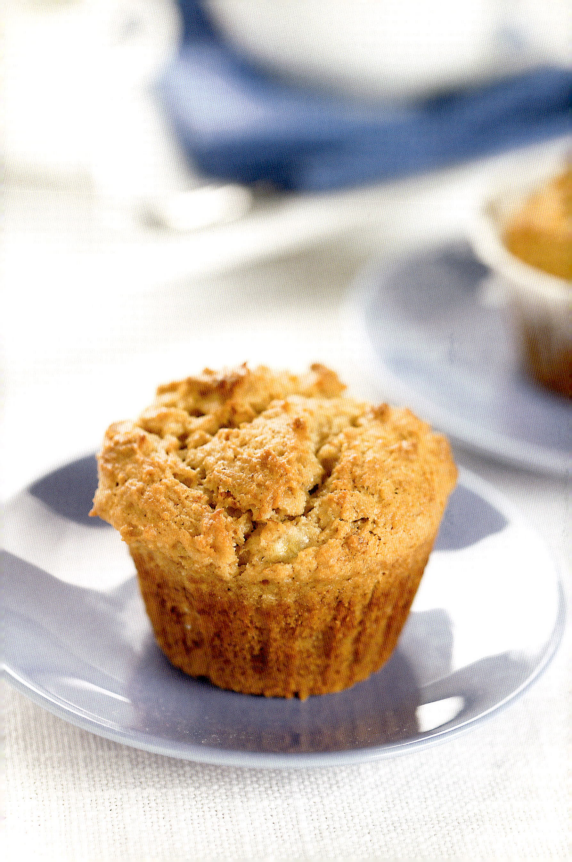

BREAKFAST QUESADILLAS

Makes 4 servings

1 cup cholesterol-free egg substitute

2 tablespoons fat-free (skim) milk

4 teaspoons canola oil, divided

1 can (4 ounces) chopped mild green chiles

8 soft corn tortillas

½ cup (2 ounces) shredded reduced-fat sharp Cheddar cheese

¼ cup chopped fresh cilantro

1 ounce turkey pepperoni slices, quartered

1 Whisk egg substitute and milk in small bowl. Heat 2 teaspoons oil in large skillet over medium heat. Cook eggs until set, lifting edges to allow uncooked portion to flow underneath. Remove from skillet. Wipe out skillet with paper towel.

2 Spread 1 tablespoon chiles on half of each tortilla. Top each with eggs, 1 tablespoon cheese and 1½ teaspoons cilantro; sprinkle evenly with pepperoni. Fold tortillas in half.

3 Heat remaining 2 teaspoons oil in skillet. Cook quesadillas in two batches 3 minutes per side or until cheese is melted.

Nutrition Information (per serving)

Calories 230, **Total Fat** 8g, **Saturated Fat** 1g, **Cholesterol** 10mg, **Sodium** 460mg, **Carbohydrates** 25g, **Dietary Fiber** 0g, **Protein** 15g

Dietary Exchanges: 1½ Bread/Starch • 1½ Meat • 1 Fat

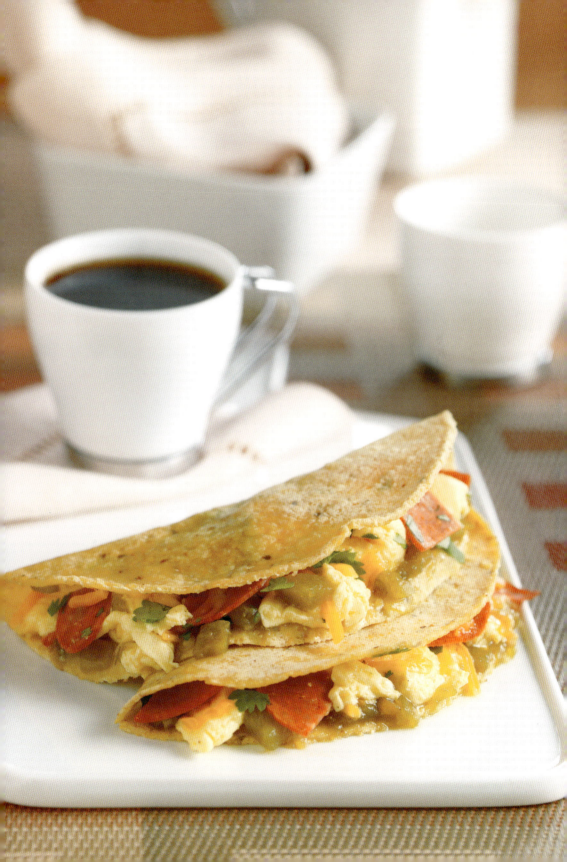

PEACH-ALMOND SCONES

Makes 12 scones

2 cups all-purpose flour

¼ cup plus 1 tablespoon sugar, divided

2 teaspoons baking powder

½ teaspoon salt

5 tablespoons cold butter or margarine

½ cup sliced almonds, toasted and divided*

1 egg

2 tablespoons reduced-fat (2%) milk

1 can (16 ounces) peach halves or slices in juice, drained and finely chopped

½ teaspoon almond extract

To toast almonds, spread in single layer on baking sheet. Bake in preheated 350°F oven 8 to 10 minutes or until golden brown, stirring frequently.

1 Preheat oven to 425°F.

2 Combine flour, ¼ cup sugar, baking powder and salt in large bowl. Cut in margarine with pastry blender or two knives until coarse crumbs form. Stir in ¼ cup almonds. Lightly beat egg and milk in small bowl. Reserve 2 tablespoons egg mixture. Stir peaches and almond extract into remaining egg mixture. Stir into flour mixture until soft dough forms.

3 Gently knead dough on floured work surface 10 to 12 times. Roll dough into 9×6-inch rectangle. Using floured knife, cut into six 3-inch squares. Cut diagonally into halves, making 12 triangles. Place 2 inches apart on ungreased baking sheets. Brush with reserved egg mixture. Sprinkle with remaining ¼ cup almonds and 1 tablespoon sugar.

4 Bake 10 to 12 minutes or until golden brown. Remove to wire racks; cool 10 minutes. Serve warm.

SERVING SUGGESTION: Serve with butter or jelly, if desired.

Nutrition Information (per serving)

Calories 195, **Total Fat** 9g, **Saturated Fat** 3g, **Cholesterol** 31mg, **Sodium** 224mg, **Carbohydrates** 27g, **Dietary Fiber** 2g, **Protein** 4g

Dietary Exchanges: 1 Bread/Starch • 1 Fruit • 1½ Fat

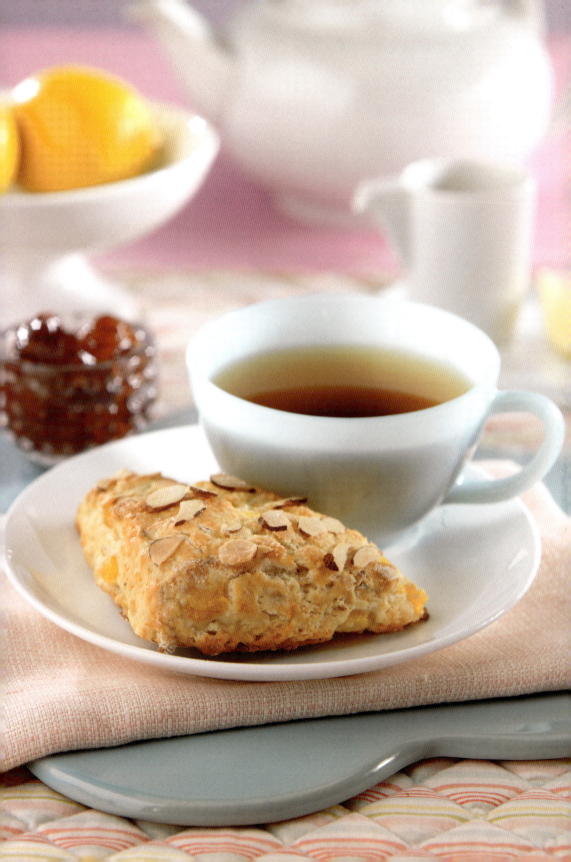

CRUSTLESS HAM AND ASPARAGUS QUICHE

Makes 6 servings

2 cups sliced asparagus (½-inch pieces)

1 red bell pepper, chopped

1 cup low-fat (1%) milk

2 tablespoons all-purpose flour

4 egg whites

1 egg

1 cup chopped cooked deli ham

2 tablespoons chopped fresh tarragon or basil

½ teaspoon salt (optional)

¼ teaspoon black pepper

½ cup (2 ounces) finely shredded Swiss cheese

1 Preheat oven to 350°F. Combine asparagus, bell pepper and 1 tablespoon water in microwavable bowl. Cover with waxed paper; microwave on HIGH 2 minutes or until vegetables are crisp-tender. Drain vegetables.

2 Whisk milk and flour in large bowl. Whisk in egg whites and egg until well combined. Stir in vegetables, ham, tarragon, salt, if desired, and black pepper. Pour into 9-inch pie plate. Bake 35 minutes. Sprinkle cheese over quiche; bake 5 minutes or until center is set and cheese is melted. Let stand 5 minutes before serving. Cut into six wedges.

VARIATIONS: Add 1 clove minced garlic. Add 2 tablespoons chopped green onion.

Nutrition Information (per serving)

Calories 138, **Total Fat** 6g, **Saturated Fat** 3g, **Cholesterol** 25mg, **Sodium** 439mg, **Carbohydrates** 8g, **Dietary Fiber** 1g, **Protein** 13g

Dietary Exchanges: 1½ Meat • 1½ Vegetable • ½ Fat

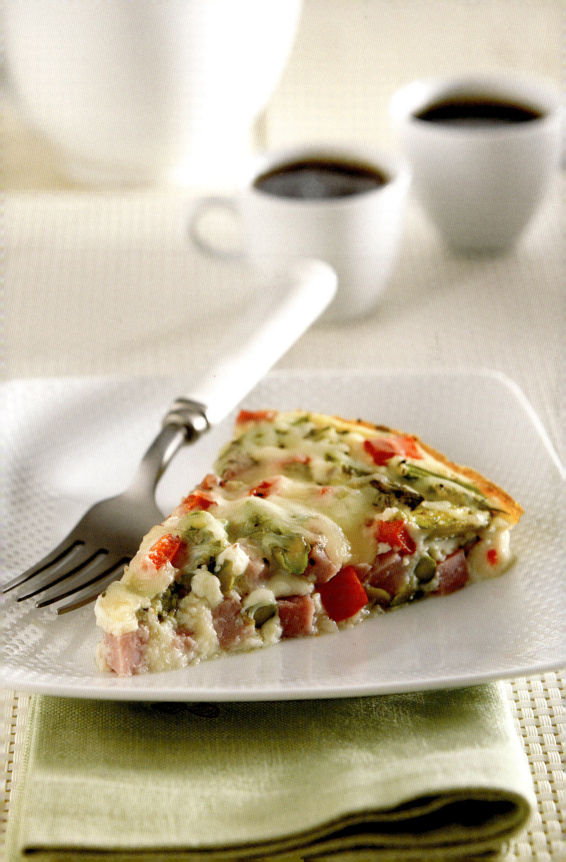

SWEET & SAVORY BREAKFAST MUFFINS

Makes 12 muffins

1¼ cups original pancake and baking mix

1 cup fat-free (skim) milk

3 egg whites

¼ cup maple syrup

4 small fully cooked turkey breakfast sausage links, diced

1 cup fresh blueberries

1 Preheat oven to 375°F. Spray 12 standard (2½-inch) muffin cups with nonstick cooking spray.

2 Stir pancake mix, milk, egg whites and maple syrup in large bowl until smooth and well blended. Fold in sausage and blueberries. Pour evenly into prepared muffin cups.

3 Bake 18 to 20 minutes or until toothpick inserted into centers comes out clean. Serve warm.

Nutrition Information (per serving)

Calories 99, **Total Fat** 2g, **Saturated Fat** 1g, **Cholesterol** 7mg, **Sodium** 232mg, **Carbohydrates** 16g, **Dietary Fiber** 1g, **Protein** 4g

Dietary Exchanges: 1 Bread/Starch • ½ Fat

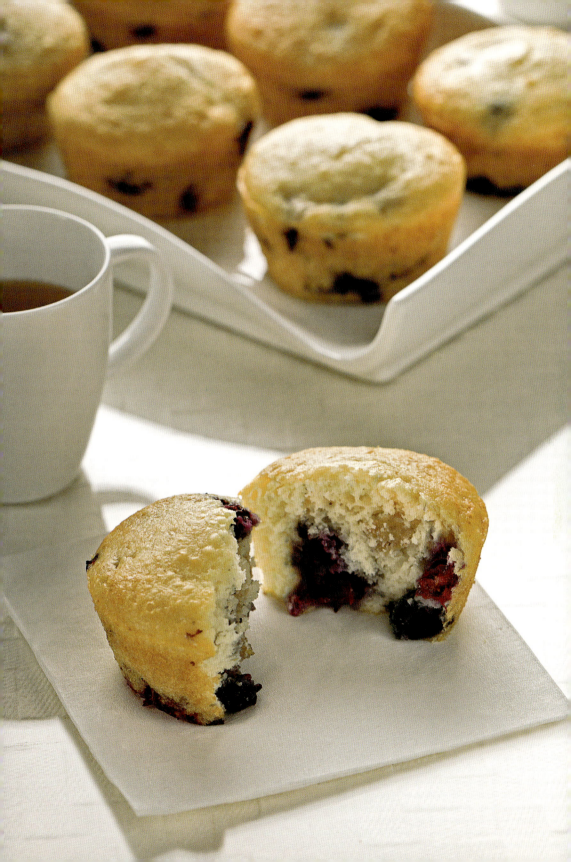

CRANBERRY BUTTERMILK PANCAKES

Makes 18 (3-inch) pancakes (about 6 servings)

1 cup all-purpose flour

1 cup whole wheat flour

2 teaspoons baking powder

1 teaspoon baking soda

½ teaspoon ground cinnamon

¼ teaspoon ground nutmeg

⅔ cup whole berry cranberry sauce, divided

2 eggs

2 tablespoons vegetable oil

1½ cups low-fat buttermilk

Sugar-free maple syrup (optional)

1 Combine all-purpose flour, whole wheat flour, baking powder, baking soda, cinnamon and nutmeg in small bowl; mix well. Whisk cranberry sauce, eggs and oil in large bowl until well blended. Gradually stir in flour mixture until combined. Stir in buttermilk until smooth and well blended.

2 Heat large nonstick griddle or skillet over medium heat. Pour ¼ cupfuls of batter 2 inches apart onto griddle. Cook 3 minutes or until lightly browned and edges begin to bubble. Turn over; cook 3 minutes or until lightly browned. Repeat with remaining batter. Serve with syrup, if desired.

Nutrition Information (per serving)

Calories 283, **Total Fat** 7g, **Saturated Fat** 2g, **Cholesterol** 64mg, **Sodium** 466mg, **Carbohydrates** 44g, **Dietary Fiber** 3g, **Protein** 9g

Dietary Exchanges: 3 Bread/Starch • 1½ Fat

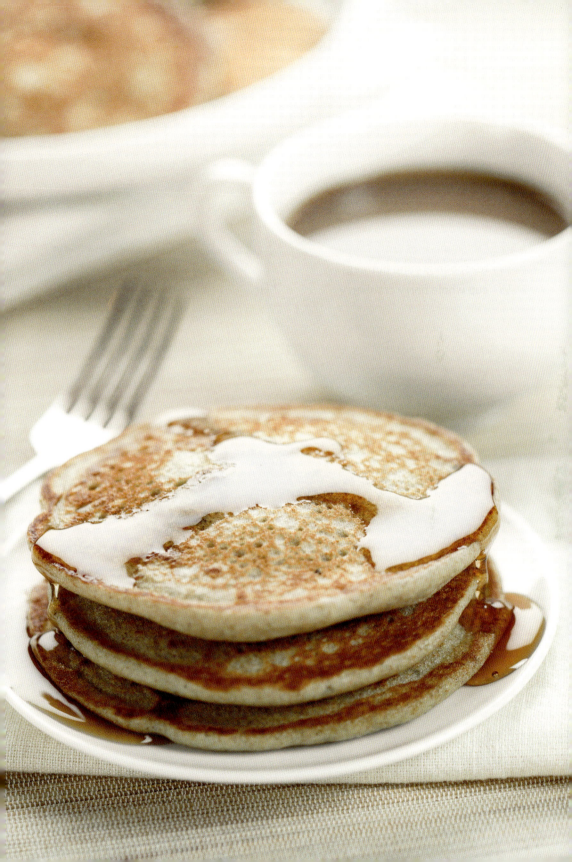

BREAKFAST PIZZA MARGHERITA

Makes 6 servings

1 (12-inch) prepared pizza crust

3 slices 95% fat-free turkey bacon

2 cups cholesterol-free egg substitute

½ cup fat-free (skim) milk

1½ tablespoons chopped fresh basil, divided

⅛ teaspoon black pepper

2 plum tomatoes, thinly sliced

½ cup (2 ounces) shredded reduced-fat mozzarella cheese

¼ cup (1 ounce) shredded reduced-fat Cheddar cheese

1 Preheat oven to 450°F. Place pizza crust on 12-inch pizza pan. Bake 6 to 8 minutes or until heated through.

2 Meanwhile, coat large skillet with nonstick cooking spray. Cook bacon over medium-high heat until crisp. Remove from skillet to paper towels; cool. Crumble bacon.

3 Combine egg substitute, milk, ½ tablespoon basil and pepper in medium bowl. Coat same skillet with cooking spray. Add egg substitute mixture. Cook over medium heat until mixture begins to set around edges. Gently stir eggs, allowing uncooked portions to flow underneath. Repeat stirring of egg mixture every 1 to 2 minutes or until eggs are just set. Remove from heat.

4 Arrange tomato slices on warmed pizza crust. Spoon scrambled eggs over tomatoes. Sprinkle with bacon. Top with cheeses. Bake 1 minute or until cheese is melted. Sprinkle with remaining 1 tablespoon basil. Cut into six wedges. Serve immediately.

Nutrition Information (per serving)

Calories 311, **Total Fat** 9g, **Saturated Fat** 2g, **Cholesterol** 11mg, **Sodium** 675mg, **Carbohydrates** 35g, **Dietary Fiber** 2g, **Protein** 21g

Dietary Exchanges: 2 Bread/Starch • 2 Meat • ½ Vegetable • 1½ Fat

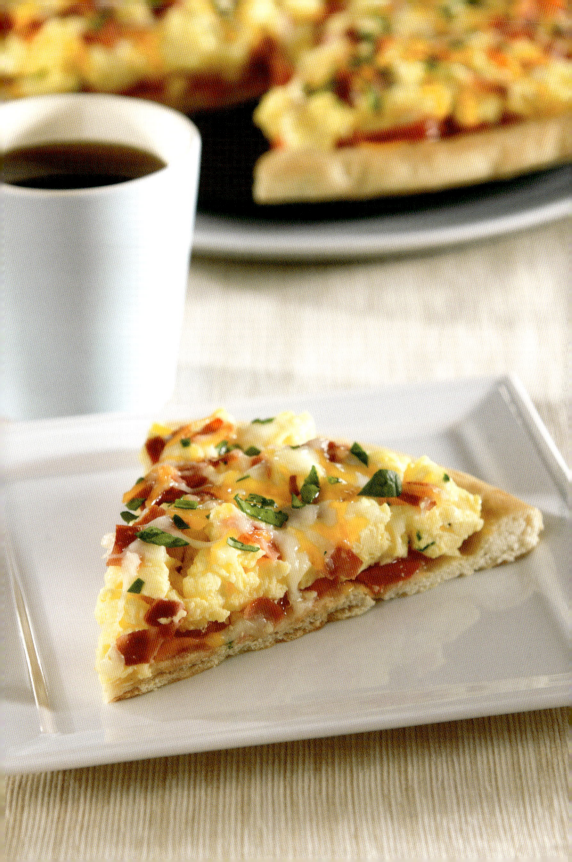

VERY BERRY YOGURT PARFAITS

Makes 4 servings

3 cups plain nonfat yogurt

2 tablespoons sugar-free berry preserves

1 packet sugar substitute*

½ teaspoon vanilla

2 cups sliced fresh strawberries

1 cup fresh blueberries

4 tablespoons sliced toasted almonds

This recipe was tested with sucralose-based sugar substitute.

1 Combine yogurt, preserves, sugar substitute and vanilla in medium bowl.

2 Layer ½ cup yogurt mixture, ¼ cup strawberries, ¼ cup blueberries and ¼ cup yogurt mixture in each of four dessert dishes. Top each parfait with remaining ¼ cup strawberries and 1 tablespoon almonds. Serve immediately.

NOTES: These parfaits would also be delicious topped with low-fat granola. Or, try another flavor of preserves for a simple variation.

Nutrition Information (per serving)

Calories 179, **Total Fat** 3g, **Saturated Fat** 1g, **Cholesterol** 4mg, **Sodium** 104mg, **Carbohydrates** 33g, **Dietary Fiber** 3g, **Protein** 10g

Dietary Exchanges: 1½ Fruit • 1 Milk

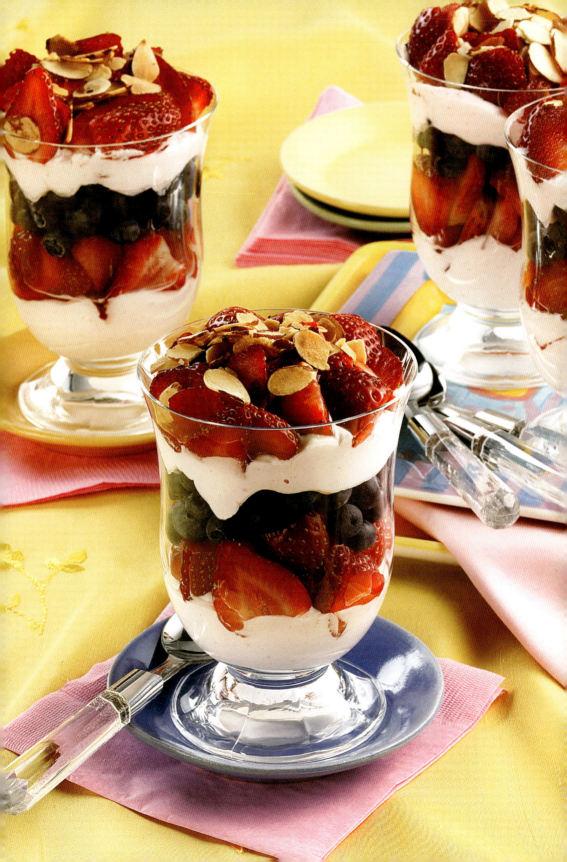

QUICK BREAKFAST BLINTZES

Makes 4 servings (2 blintzes per serving)

1 teaspoon unsalted butter

¼ teaspoon ground cinnamon, plus additional for serving

¼ teaspoon ground nutmeg

2 ripe but firm Bartlett pears, peeled and cut into ½-inch cubes

1 teaspoon vanilla

1½ cups reduced-fat ricotta cheese

8 (8-inch) packaged thin crêpes

3 teaspoons powdered sugar, divided

1 Melt butter in 10-inch nonstick skillet over medium heat. Stir ¼ teaspoon cinnamon and nutmeg into butter. Add pears; cook and stir 3 to 4 minutes or until warmed and tender.

2 Add vanilla to ricotta cheese in small bowl; stir well. Place crêpes on sheet of waxed paper sprinkled with 1 teaspoon powdered sugar. Spoon ricotta cheese mixture down center of crêpes. Spoon pears over cheese; roll up and place on microwave-safe serving plates.

3 Microwave each serving separately on HIGH 20 to 30 seconds or until warm.

4 Place remaining 2 teaspoons powdered sugar in fine mesh strainer; shake over crêpes. Sprinkle with additional cinnamon, if desired.

Nutrition Information (per serving)

Calories 231, **Total Fat** 6g, **Saturated Fat** 3g, **Cholesterol** 35mg, **Sodium** 183mg, **Carbohydrates** 34g, **Dietary Fiber** 4g, **Protein** 10g

Dietary Exchanges: 2 Bread/Starch • ½ Meat • ½ Fruit • ½ Fat

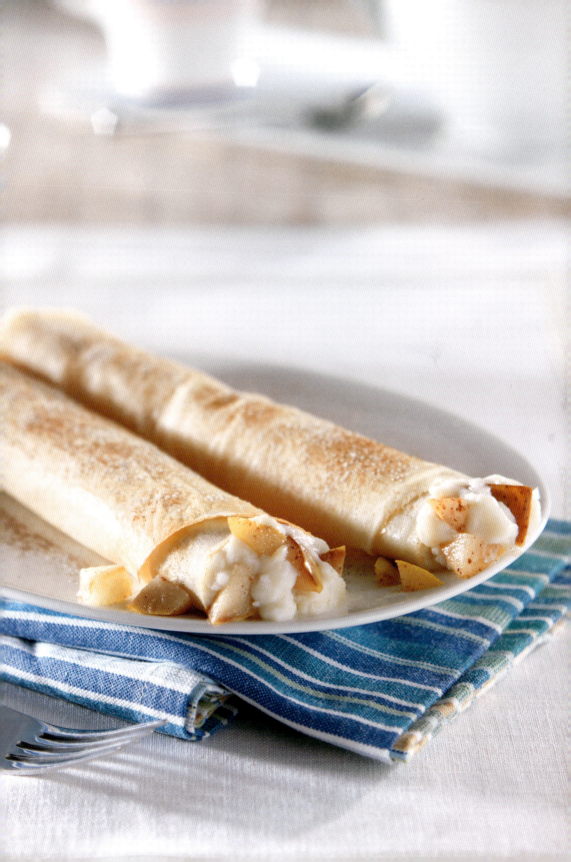

CARROT-PECAN MUFFINS

Makes 18 muffins

1 cup all-purpose flour

1 cup whole wheat flour

2 teaspoons baking powder

2 teaspoons ground cinnamon

1 teaspoon baking soda

¼ teaspoon salt

⅛ teaspoon ground cloves

2 eggs, lightly beaten

1 cup packed brown sugar

½ cup fat-free (skim) milk

¼ cup canola oil

¼ cup natural or unsweetened applesauce

1 teaspoon vanilla

2 cups finely shredded carrots

⅓ cup chopped pecans

1 Preheat oven to 375°F. Line 18 standard (2½-inch) muffin cups with paper baking cups or spray with nonstick cooking spray.

2 Combine all-purpose flour, whole wheat flour, baking powder, cinnamon, baking soda, salt and cloves in large bowl; mix well. Whisk eggs and brown sugar in medium bowl until combined. Stir in milk, oil, applesauce and vanilla until smooth. Stir into flour mixture until combined. Fold in carrots and pecans. Spoon mixture evenly into prepared muffin cups.

3 Bake 18 to 20 minutes or until toothpick inserted into centers comes out clean. Cool in pans 5 minutes. Remove to wire racks; cool completely.

Nutrition Information (per serving)

Calories 154, **Total Fat** 5g, **Saturated Fat** 1g, **Cholesterol** 21mg, **Sodium** 180mg, **Carbohydrates** 25g, **Dietary Fiber** 2g, **Protein** 3g

Dietary Exchanges: 1½ Bread/Starch • 1 Fat

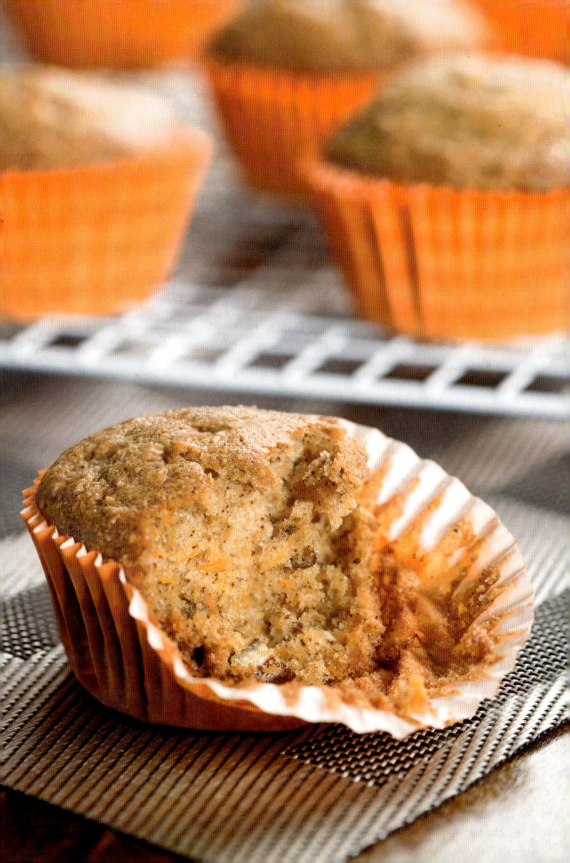

WHOLE GRAIN FRENCH TOAST

Makes 4 servings (2 slices toast and ¼ cup blueberry mixture per serving)

½   cup egg substitute *or* 2 egg whites

¼   cup low-fat (1%) milk

½   teaspoon ground cinnamon

¼   teaspoon ground nutmeg

4   teaspoons butter

8   slices 100% whole wheat or multigrain bread

⅓   cup pure maple syrup

1   cup fresh blueberries

2   teaspoons powdered sugar

1 Preheat oven to 400°F. Spray baking sheet with nonstick cooking spray.

2 Whisk egg substitute, milk, cinnamon and nutmeg in shallow bowl until well blended. Melt 1 teaspoon butter in large nonstick skillet over medium heat. Working with two slices at a time, dip each bread slice in milk mixture, turning to coat both sides; let excess mixture drip back into bowl. Cook 2 minutes per side or until golden brown. Transfer to prepared baking sheet. Repeat with remaining butter, bread and milk mixture.

3 Bake 5 to 6 minutes or until heated through.

4 Microwave maple syrup in small microwavable bowl on HIGH 30 seconds or until bubbly. Stir in blueberries. Place french toast on four serving plates; top evenly with blueberry mixture. Sprinkle with powdered sugar.

Nutrition Information (per serving)

Calories 251, **Total Fat** 6g, **Saturated Fat** 3g, **Cholesterol** 11mg, **Sodium** 324mg, **Carbohydrates** 46g, **Dietary Fiber** 5g, **Protein** 12g

Dietary Exchanges: 2 Bread/Starch • 1 Meat • 1 Fruit

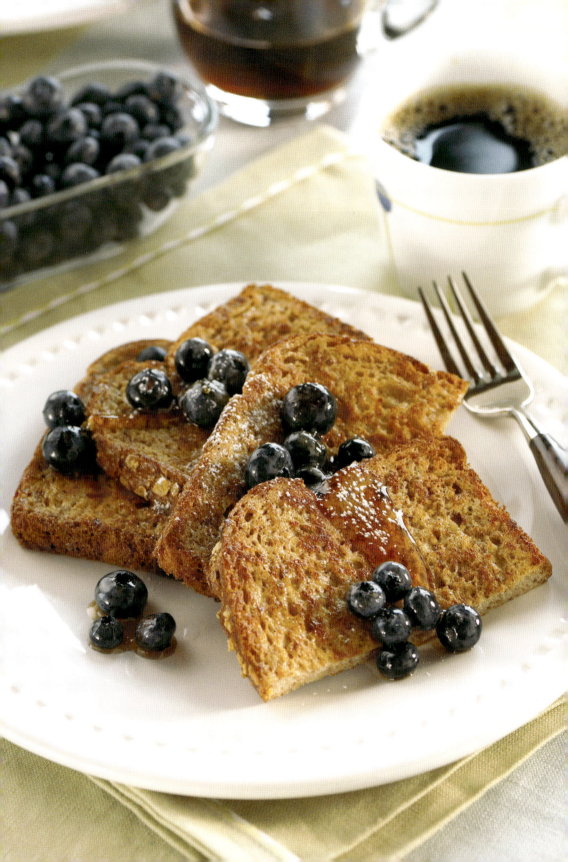

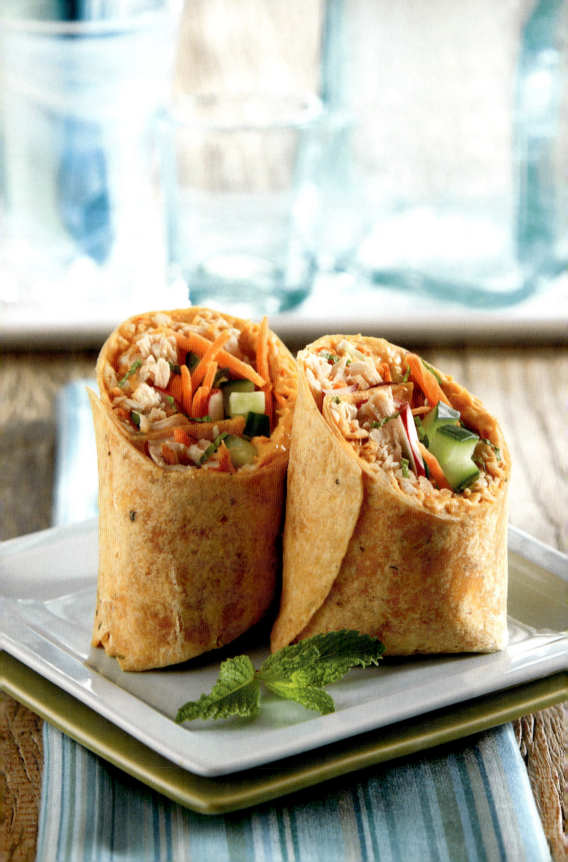

CHICKEN, HUMMUS AND VEGETABLE WRAPS

Makes 4 servings (1 wrap per serving)

¾ **cup hummus (regular, roasted red pepper or roasted garlic)**

4 **(8- to 10-inch) sun-dried tomato *or* spinach wraps *or* whole wheat tortillas**

2 **cups chopped cooked chicken breast**

Chipotle hot pepper sauce *or* Louisiana-style hot pepper sauce (optional)

½ **cup shredded carrots**

½ **cup chopped unpeeled cucumber**

½ **cup thinly sliced radishes**

2 **tablespoons chopped fresh mint *or* basil**

Spread hummus evenly over wraps all the way to edges. Arrange chicken over hummus; sprinkle with hot pepper sauce, if desired. Top with carrots, cucumber, radishes and mint. Roll up tightly. Cut in half diagonally.

VARIATION: Substitute alfalfa sprouts for the radishes. For tasty appetizers, cut wraps into bite-size pieces.

Nutrition Information (per serving)

Calories 308, **Total Fat** 10g, **Saturated Fat** 1g, **Cholesterol** 60mg, **Sodium** 540mg, **Carbohydrates** 32g, **Dietary Fiber** 15g, **Protein** 32g

Dietary Exchanges: 2 Bread/Starch • 3 Meat

GINGERED BBQ'D SHRIMP SKEWERS

Makes 6 servings (2 skewers per serving)

¼ cup bottled barbecue sauce

¼ cup no-sugar-added raspberry fruit spread

1 tablespoon grated fresh ginger

1½ tablespoons balsamic vinegar

⅛ teaspoon red pepper flakes

24 medium raw shrimp, peeled and deveined (with tails on)

4 bacon slices, each cut into 6 pieces

12 green onions, green part only, cut in half (24 pieces total)

1 can (12 ounces) pineapple chunks, drained

12 (6-inch) bamboo skewers, soaked in water

1 Preheat grill to medium-high heat.

2 Coat cold grid with nonstick cooking spray; place over heat.

3 In small bowl, combine barbecue sauce, fruit spread, ginger, vinegar and red pepper flakes. Whisk until well blended; set aside.

4 Thread skewers with 2 shrimp, 2 bacon pieces, 2 green onion pieces and 2 pineapple chunks per skewer.

5 Place half of sauce in separate bowl; set aside.

6 Place skewers on grid, baste with remaining sauce; grill 3 minutes total or until shrimp are pink and opaque, turning and basting frequently. Remove from heat, baste with reserved sauce.

Nutrition Information (per serving)

Calories 115, **Total Fat** 3g, **Saturated Fat** 1g, **Cholesterol** 47mg, **Sodium** 270mg, **Carbohydrates** 13g, **Dietary Fiber** 1g, **Protein** 8g

Dietary Exchanges: 1 Bread/Starch • 1 Meat

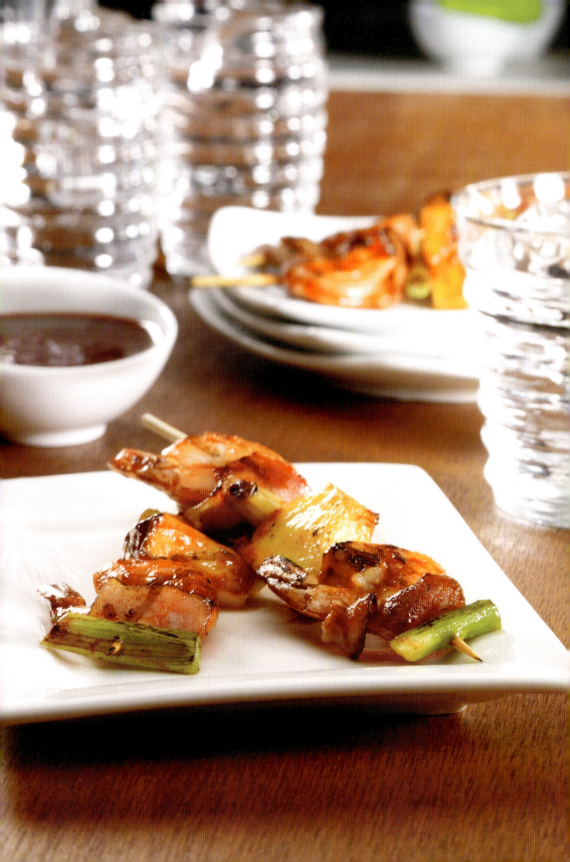

MEDITERRANEAN TUNA CUPS

Makes 10 servings (3 tuna cups per serving)

3   English cucumbers

⅔   cup plain nonfat Greek yogurt

⅓   cup coarsely chopped pitted
       kalamata olives

⅓   cup finely chopped red onion

2   tablespoons fresh lemon juice

¼   teaspoon garlic salt

2   cans (5 ounces each) solid
       white albacore tuna in water,
       drained and flaked

1 Cut ends off of each cucumber; cut each cucumber into 10 slices. Scoop out cucumber slices with a rounded ½ teaspoon, leaving thick shell.

2 Stir yogurt, olives, onion, lemon juice and garlic salt in large bowl until smooth and well blended. Stir in tuna.

3 Spoon about 1 tablespoon tuna salad into each cucumber cup. Serve immediately.

Nutrition Information (per serving)

Calories 32, **Total Fat** 1g, **Saturated Fat** 0g, **Cholesterol** 8mg, **Sodium** 102mg, **Carbohydrates** 2g, **Dietary Fiber** 1g, **Protein** 5g

Dietary Exchanges: 1 Meat

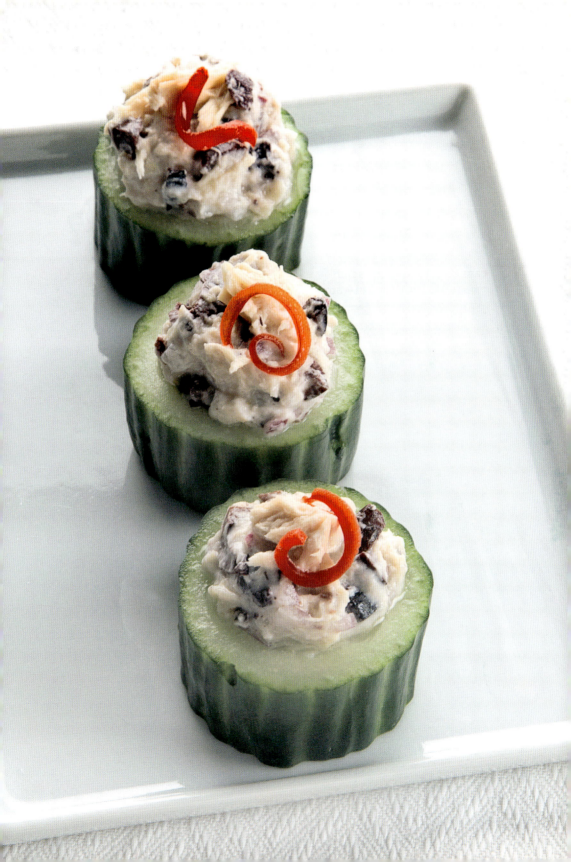

TURKEY MEATBALLS IN CRANBERRY-BARBECUE SAUCE

Makes 12 servings (2 meatballs and 2 tablespoons sauce per serving)

1   can (16 ounces) jellied cranberry sauce

½   cup barbecue sauce

1   egg white

1   pound ground turkey

1   green onion, sliced

2   teaspoons grated orange peel

1   teaspoon soy sauce

¼   teaspoon black pepper

⅛   teaspoon ground red pepper (optional)

SLOW COOKER DIRECTIONS

1 Combine cranberry sauce and barbecue sauce in slow cooker. Cover; cook on HIGH 20 to 30 minutes or until cranberry sauce is melted and mixture is heated through.

2 Meanwhile, beat egg white in medium bowl. Add turkey, green onion, orange peel, soy sauce, black pepper and ground red pepper, if desired; mix well. Shape into 24 balls.

3 Spray large nonstick skillet with nonstick cooking spray; heat over medium heat. Add meatballs; cook 8 to 10 minutes or until browned on all sides. Add to slow cooker; stir gently to coat with sauce mixture.

4 Turn slow cooker to LOW. Cover; cook 3 hours. Serve warm.

Nutrition Information (per serving)

Calories 137, **Total Fat** 4g, **Saturated Fat** 1g, **Cholesterol** 19mg, **Sodium** 206mg, **Carbohydrates** 18g, **Dietary Fiber** 1g, **Protein** 7g

Dietary Exchanges: 1 Meat • 1 Fruit • ½ Fat

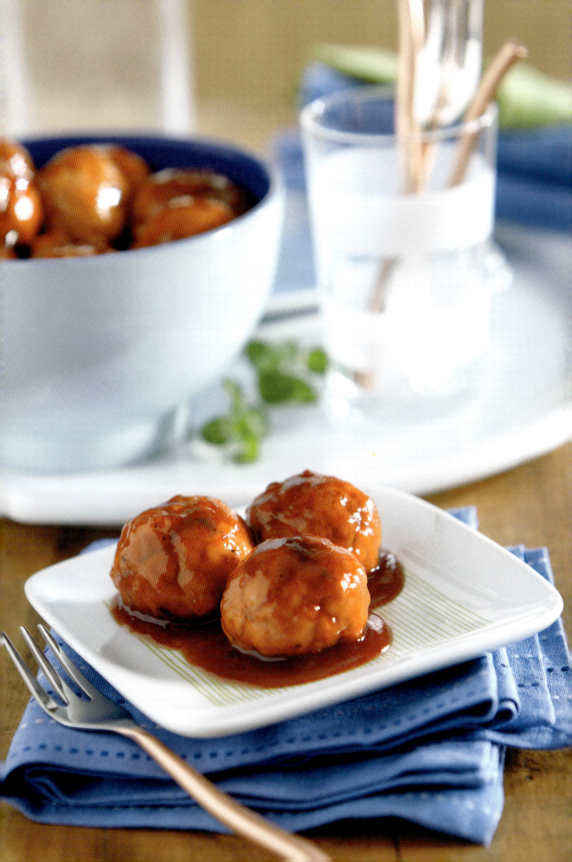

ONION AND SHRIMP FLATBREAD PIZZA WITH GOAT CHEESE

Makes 6 servings (2 pieces per serving)

4   teaspoons olive oil, divided

3   large onions, thinly sliced

¼   teaspoon salt

1   container (about 14 ounces) refrigerated pizza dough

½   pound small raw shrimp, peeled

⅛   cup chopped fresh chives

3   ounces goat cheese, crumbled

½   teaspoon black pepper (optional)

1 Heat 2 teaspoons oil in large skillet over medium heat. Add onions; cook and stir about 8 minutes. Stir in salt. Reduce heat to medium-low; cook 25 minutes or until onions are soft and deep golden brown, stirring occasionally. If onions are cooking too quickly, reduce heat to low.

2 Meanwhile, preheat oven to 425°F. Roll out dough on 15×10-inch baking sheet. Bake 8 to 10 minutes or until crust is golden brown. Turn off oven. Spread caramelized onions over crust.

3 Heat remaining 2 teaspoons oil in same skillet over medium heat. Add shrimp; cook and stir 2 minutes or until pink and opaque. Arrange shrimp over onions on pizza; sprinkle with chives, goat cheese and pepper, if desired.

4 Place pizza in warm oven 1 to 2 minutes or until cheese is soft. Cut into 12 squares.

Nutrition Information (per serving)

Calories 281, **Total Fat** 8g, **Saturated Fat** 3g, **Cholesterol** 63mg, **Sodium** 677mg, **Carbohydrates** 38g, **Dietary Fiber** 2g, **Protein** 14g

Dietary Exchanges: 2 Bread/Starch • 1 Meat • 1 Vegetable • 1 Fat

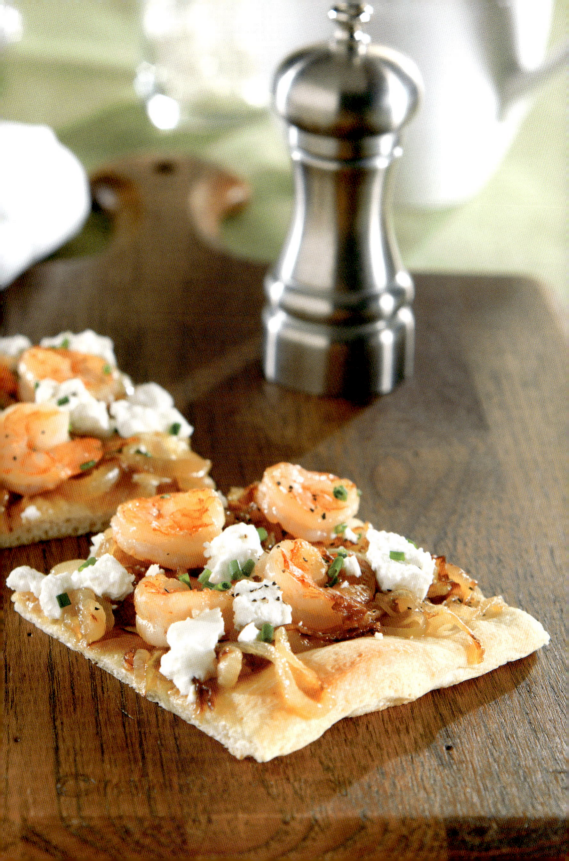

TERIYAKI CHICKEN DRUMMIES

Makes 12 servings (2 drummettes per serving)

1 bottle (10 ounces) low-sodium teriyaki sauce, divided

4 cloves garlic, crushed

1/4 teaspoon black pepper

3 pounds chicken drummettes (about 24 pieces total)

1 tablespoon toasted sesame seeds*

*To toast sesame seeds, spread seeds in small skillet. Shake skillet over medium-low heat about 3 minutes or until seeds begin to pop and turn golden.

1 Reserve 1/4 cup teriyaki sauce; set aside. Combine remaining teriyaki sauce, garlic and pepper in shallow baking dish. Add drummettes; marinate in refrigerator for 30 minutes, turning once.

2 Preheat oven to 400°F. Spray baking sheet with nonstick cooking spray. Remove drummettes from dish; discard marinade. Place drummettes, skin side up, on prepared baking sheet.

3 Bake 30 minutes or until golden brown. Immediately remove drummettes to large bowl. Add reserved 1/4 cup teriyaki sauce; toss to coat evenly. Sprinkle with sesame seeds.

Nutrition Information (per serving)

Calories 160, **Total Fat** 10g, **Saturated Fat** 2g, **Cholesterol** 40mg, **Sodium** 300mg, **Carbohydrates** 2g, **Dietary Fiber** 0g, **Protein** 12g

Dietary Exchanges: 1½ Meat • 1½ Fat

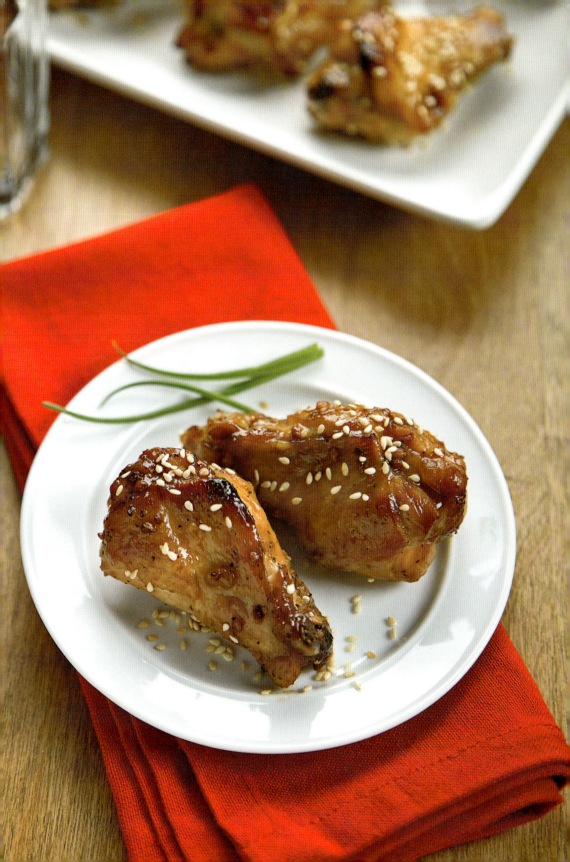

TUNA CAKES WITH CREAMY CUCUMBER SAUCE

Makes 5 servings (1 tuna cake and 2 tablespoons sauce per serving)

½ cup finely chopped cucumber

½ cup fat-free plain yogurt or fat-free plain Greek yogurt

1½ teaspoons chopped fresh dill or ½ teaspoon dried dill weed

1 teaspoon lemon-pepper seasoning

⅓ cup shredded carrots

¼ cup sliced green onions

¼ cup finely chopped celery

¼ cup reduced-fat mayonnaise

2 teaspoons spicy brown mustard

1 cup panko bread crumbs, divided

1 can (12 ounces) albacore tuna in water, drained

3 teaspoons canola oil or olive oil, divided

Lemon wedges (optional)

1 For sauce, stir together cucumber, yogurt, dill and lemon-pepper seasoning in small bowl. Cover and refrigerate until serving time.

2 In mixing bowl, combine carrots, green onions, celery, mayonnaise and mustard. Stir in ½ cup panko. Add tuna and mix until combined.

3 Place remaining ½ cup panko in shallow dish. Shape tuna mixture into 5 (½-inch-thick) patties. Dip patties in panko, lightly coating.

4 Heat 1½ teaspoons oil in 10-inch nonstick skillet. Add patties. Cook, uncovered, over medium heat 5 to 6 minutes or until golden brown, turning once. Add remaining 1½ teaspoons oil to skillet when patties are turned. Serve with yogurt mixture and garnish with lemon wedges, if desired.

Nutrition Information (per serving)

Calories 200, **Total Fat** 8g, **Saturated Fat** 1g, **Cholesterol** 35mg, **Sodium** 310mg, **Carbohydrates** 14g, **Dietary Fiber** 0g, **Protein** 18g

Dietary Exchanges: 1 Bread/Starch • 2 Meat • ½ Vegetable • 1 ½ Fat

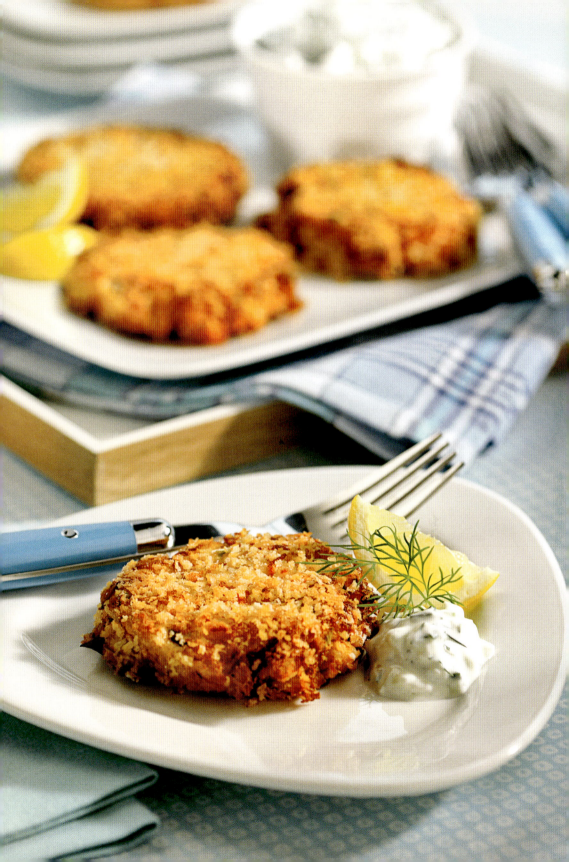

ROASTED EGGPLANT ROLLS

Makes 8 servings (2 rolls per serving)

2   medium eggplants (¾ pound each)

2   tablespoons lemon juice

1   teaspoon olive oil

4   tablespoons (2 ounces) fat-free cream cheese

2   tablespoons fat-free sour cream

1   green onion, minced

4   sun-dried tomatoes (packed in oil), rinsed, drained and minced

1   clove garlic, minced

¼   teaspoon dried oregano

⅛   teaspoon black pepper

16 fresh stemmed spinach leaves

1   cup meatless pasta sauce

1 Preheat oven to 450°F. Spray two nonstick baking sheets with nonstick cooking spray; set aside. Trim ends from eggplants. Cut eggplants lengthwise into ¼-inch-thick slices. Discard outside slices that are mostly skin. (You will have about 16 slices total.) Arrange slices in single layer on prepared baking sheets.

2 Combine lemon juice and oil in small bowl; brush lightly over both sides of eggplant slices. Bake 22 to 24 minutes or until slightly golden brown, turning once. Transfer eggplant slices to plate; cool.

3 Meanwhile, stir together cream cheese, sour cream, green onion, sun-dried tomatoes, garlic, oregano and pepper in small bowl until blended.

4 Spread about 1 teaspoon cream cheese mixture evenly over each eggplant slice. Arrange spinach leaf on top, leaving ½-inch border. Roll up, beginning at small end. Lay rolls, seam side down, on serving platter. (If making ahead, cover and refrigerate up to 2 days. Bring to room temperature before serving.) Serve with warmed pasta sauce.

Nutrition Information (per serving)

Calories 77, **Total Fat** 3g, **Saturated Fat** 1g, **Cholesterol** 0mg, **Sodium** 213mg, **Carbohydrates** 12g, **Dietary Fiber** 1g, **Protein** 3g

Dietary Exchanges: 2 Vegetable • ½ Fat

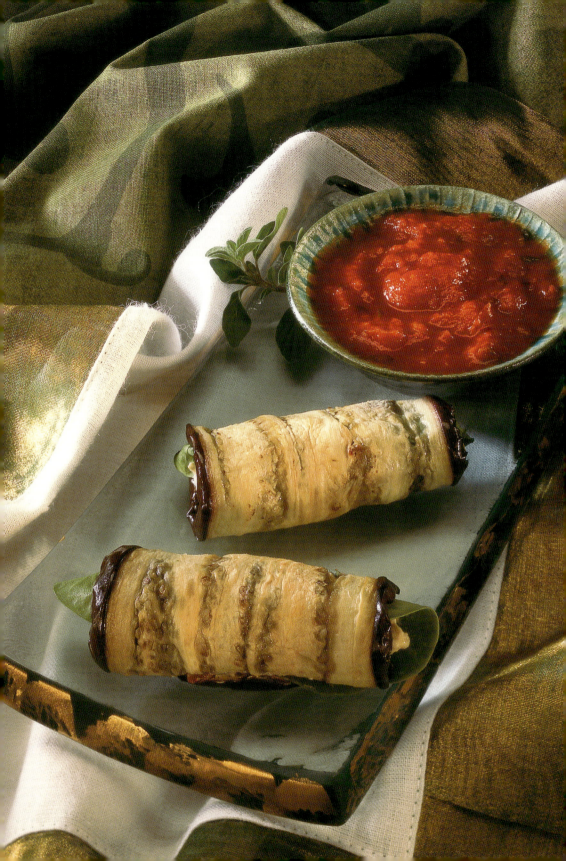

MINI MARINATED BEEF SKEWERS

Makes 6 servings (3 skewers per serving)

1 beef top round steak (about 1 pound)

2 tablespoons reduced-sodium soy sauce

1 tablespoon dry sherry

1 teaspoon dark sesame oil

2 cloves garlic, minced

18 cherry tomatoes, halved (optional)

1 Cut beef crosswise into 18 (1/8-inch-thick) slices. Place in large resealable food storage bag. Combine soy sauce, sherry, oil and garlic in small cup; pour over beef. Seal bag; turn to coat. Marinate in refrigerator at least 30 minutes or up to 2 hours.

2 Meanwhile, soak 18 (6-inch) wooden skewers in water 20 minutes.

3 Preheat broiler. Drain beef; discard marinade. Weave beef accordion-style onto skewers. Place on rack of broiler pan.

4 Broil 4 to 5 inches from heat 2 minutes. Turn skewers over; broil 2 minutes more or until beef is barely pink.

5 Garnish with cherry tomatoes. Serve warm.

Nutrition Information (per serving)

Calories 120, **Total Fat** 4g, **Saturated Fat** 1g, **Cholesterol** 60mg, **Sodium** 99mg, **Carbohydrates** 2g, **Dietary Fiber** 1g, **Protein** 20g

Dietary Exchanges: 2 Meat

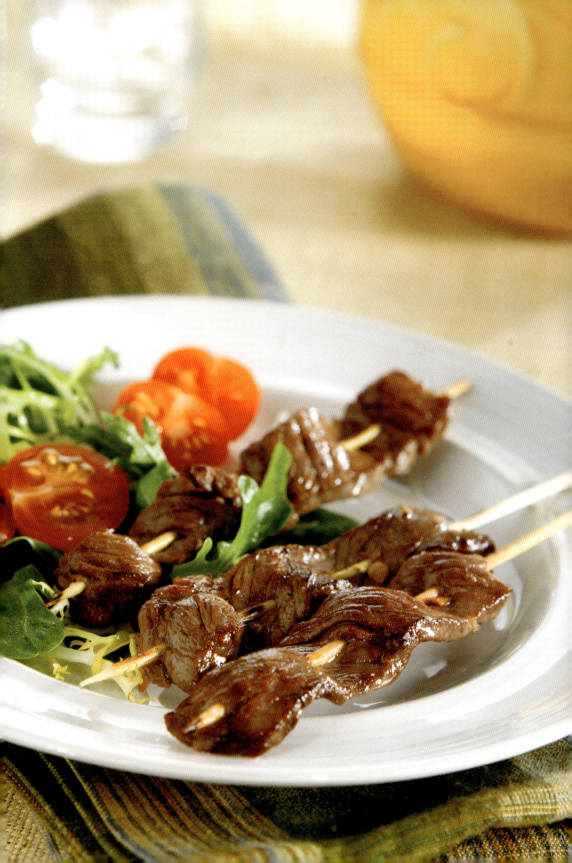

SWIMMING TUNA DIP

Makes 4 servings

1 cup low-fat (1%) cottage cheese

1 tablespoon reduced-fat mayonnaise

1 tablespoon lemon juice

2 teaspoons dry ranch-style salad dressing mix

1 can (3 ounces) chunk white tuna packed in water, drained and flaked

2 tablespoons sliced green onion or chopped celery

1 teaspoon dried parsley flakes

1 package (12 ounces) peeled baby carrots

1 Combine cottage cheese, mayonnaise, lemon juice and salad dressing mix in food processor or blender. Cover and blend until smooth.

2 Combine tuna, green onion and parsley flakes in small bowl. Stir in cottage cheese mixture. Serve with carrots.

Nutrition Information (per serving)

Calories 116, **Total Fat** 3g, **Saturated Fat** 1g, **Cholesterol** 12mg, **Sodium** 449mg, **Carbohydrates** 10g, **Dietary Fiber** 2g, **Protein** 13g

Dietary Exchanges: 2 Meat • 1 Vegetable

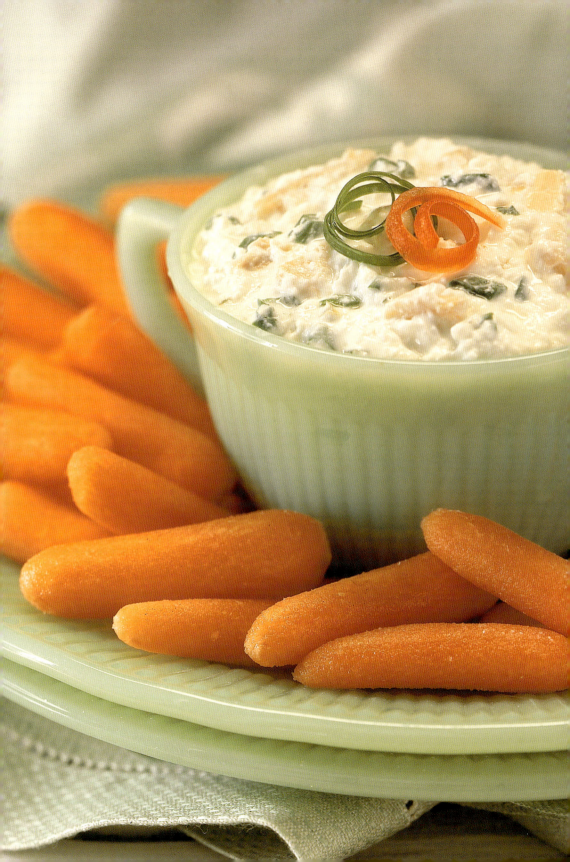

VEGGIE SUSHI ROLLS

Makes 4 servings (6 pieces per serving)

2 tablespoons unseasoned rice vinegar

1 teaspoon sugar

½ teaspoon salt

2 cups cooked short grain brown rice

4 sheets sushi nori

1 teaspoon toasted sesame seeds

½ English cucumber, cut into ¼-inch thin pieces

½ red bell pepper, cut into ¼-inch thin pieces

½ ripe avocado, cut into ½-inch thin pieces

Pickled ginger and/or wasabi paste (optional)

1 Combine vinegar, sugar and salt in large bowl. Stir in rice. Cover with damp towel until ready to use.

2 Prepare small bowl with water and splash of vinegar to rinse fingers and prevent rice from sticking while working. Place 1 sheet of nori horizontally on bamboo sushi mat or waxed or parchment paper, rough side up. Using wet fingers, spread about ½ cup rice evenly over nori, leaving 1-inch border along bottom edge. Sprinkle rice with ¼ teaspoon sesame seeds. Place one fourth of each cucumber, bell pepper and avocado on top of rice.

3 Pick up edge of mat nearest you. Roll mat forward, wrapping rice around fillings and pressing gently to form log; press gently to seal. Place roll on cutting board, seam side down. Repeat with remaining nori and fillings.

4 Slice each roll into six pieces using sharp knife.* Cut off ends, if desired. Serve with pickled ginger and/or wasabi, if desired.

Wipe knife with damp cloth between cuts, if necessary.

Nutrition Information (per serving)

Calories 165, **Total Fat** 4g, **Saturated Fat** 1g, **Cholesterol** 0mg, **Sodium** 295mg, **Carbohydrates** 29g, **Dietary Fiber** 5g, **Protein** 4g

Dietary Exchanges: 2 Bread/Starch • ½ **Fat**

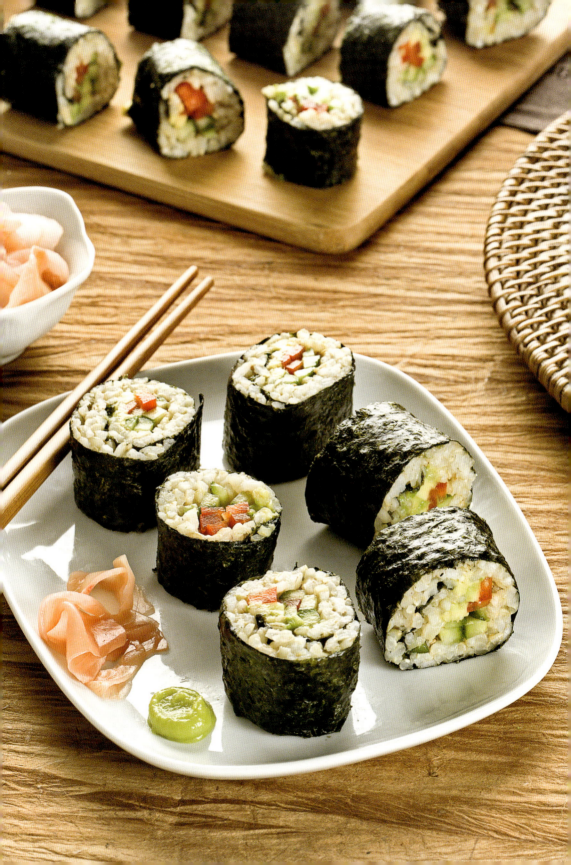

SAVORY PUMPKIN HUMMUS

Makes 1½ cups (12 [2-tablespoon] servings)

1 can (15 ounces) solid-pack pumpkin

3 tablespoons chopped fresh parsley, plus additional for garnish

3 tablespoons tahini

3 tablespoons fresh lemon juice

3 cloves garlic

1 teaspoon ground cumin

½ teaspoon salt

⅛ teaspoon black pepper

⅛ teaspoon ground red pepper, plus additional for garnish

Assorted vegetable sticks

1 Combine pumpkin, 3 tablespoons parsley, tahini, lemon juice, garlic, cumin, salt, black pepper and ⅛ teaspoon ground red pepper in food processor or blender; process until smooth. Cover and refrigerate at least 2 hours to allow flavors to develop.

2 Sprinkle with additional ground red pepper, if desired. Garnish with additional parsley. Serve with assorted vegetable sticks.

Nutrition Information (per serving)

Calories 38, **Total Fat** 2g, **Saturated Fat** 0g, **Cholesterol** 0mg, **Sodium** 101mg, **Carbohydrates** 4g, **Dietary Fiber** 1g, **Protein** 1g

Dietary Exchanges: 1 Vegetable • ½ Fat

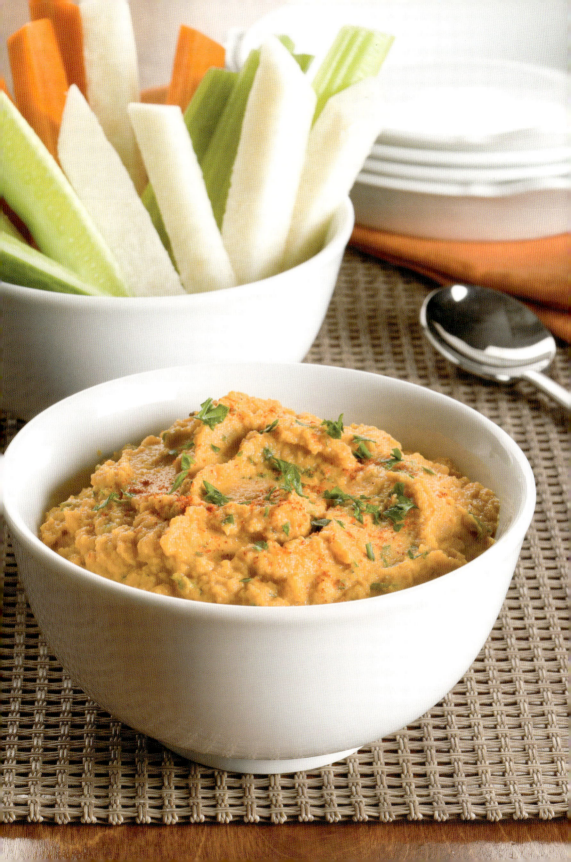

MASHED POTATO PUFFS

Makes 18 puffs (3 puffs per serving)

1 cup prepared mashed potatoes

½ cup finely chopped broccoli or spinach

2 egg whites

4 tablespoons shredded Parmesan cheese, divided

1 Preheat oven to 400°F. Spray 18 mini (1¾-inch) muffin cups with nonstick cooking spray.

2 Combine mashed potatoes, broccoli, egg whites and 2 tablespoons cheese in large bowl; mix well. Spoon evenly into prepared muffin cups. Sprinkle with remaining 2 tablespoons cheese.

3 Bake 20 to 23 minutes or until golden brown. To remove from pan, gently run knife around outer edges and lift out with fork. Serve warm.

Nutrition Information (per serving)

Calories 63, **Total Fat** 2g, **Saturated Fat** 1g, **Cholesterol** 2mg, **Sodium** 99mg, **Carbohydrates** 8g, **Dietary Fiber** 1g, **Protein** 32g

Dietary Exchanges: 1 Vegetable • ½ Fat

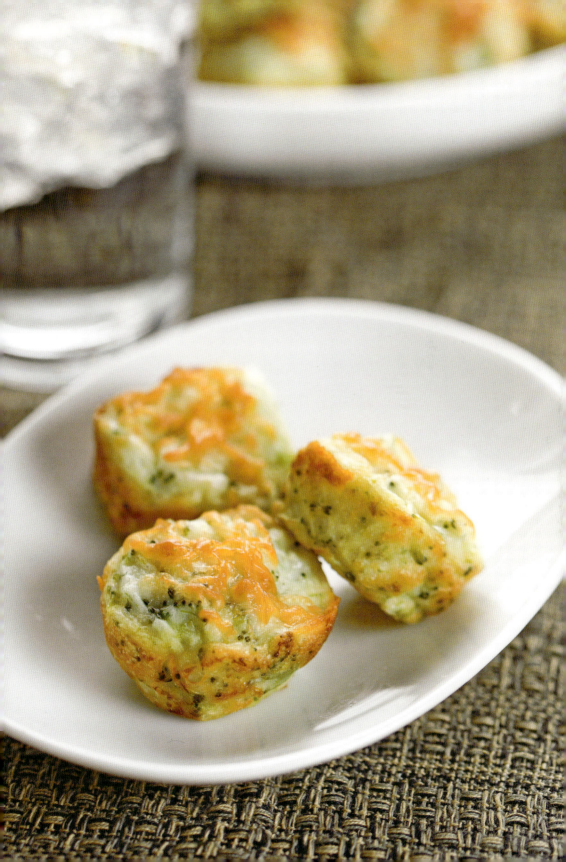

BAKED BUFFALO CHICKEN DIP

Makes 2 cups (16 [2-tablespoon] servings)

1 container (8 ounces) light cream cheese spread

¼ cup reduced-fat crumbled blue cheese

2 cups chopped cooked chicken breast (about 8 ounces)

3 tablespoons light mayonnaise

3 tablespoons light sour cream

¼ to ½ cup hot pepper sauce

1 cup (4 ounces) shredded Monterey Jack cheese

2 tablespoons panko bread crumbs

Assorted vegetable sticks and/or pita chips

1 Preheat oven to 400°F. Spray 1-quart casserole with nonstick cooking spray.

2 Combine cream cheese and blue cheese in medium saucepan; heat over medium heat until melted. Remove from heat. Stir in chicken, mayonnaise, sour cream and hot pepper sauce until combined.

3 Spread chicken mixture in prepared dish. Sprinkle with Monterey Jack cheese; top evenly with panko. Spray with cooking spray.

4 Bake 20 minutes or until lightly browned and heated through. Serve with assorted vegetable sticks and/or pita chips.

Nutrition Information (per serving)

Calories 103, **Total Fat** 6g, **Saturated Fat** 3g, **Cholesterol** 33mg, **Sodium** 226mg, **Carbohydrates** 3g, **Dietary Fiber** 0g, **Protein** 9g

Dietary Exchanges: 1 Meat • 1 Fat

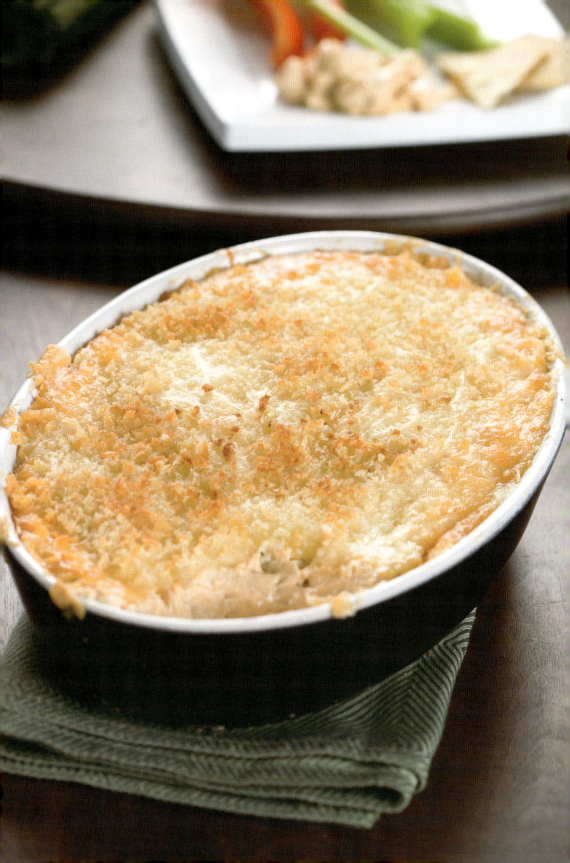

BLT LETTUCE WRAPS

Makes 8 servings (1 wrap per serving)

¼ cup plus 2 tablespoons light mayonnaise

¼ cup fat-free (skim) milk

2 teaspoons cider vinegar

¼ teaspoon garlic powder

4 cups halved grape tomatoes

16 slices center-cut bacon, crisp cooked and chopped

1 cup small croutons

8 small butter lettuce leaves

1 Whisk mayonnaise, milk, vinegar and garlic powder in small bowl until smooth and well blended.

2 Arrange tomatoes, bacon and croutons evenly on lettuce leaves. Drizzle with dressing. Serve immediately.

Nutrition Information (per serving)

Calories 112, **Total Fat** 7g, **Saturated Fat** 2g, **Cholesterol** 17mg, **Sodium** 388mg, **Carbohydrates** 8g, **Dietary Fiber** 1g, **Protein** 6g

Dietary Exchanges: ½ Bread/Starch • ½ Meat • 1 Fat

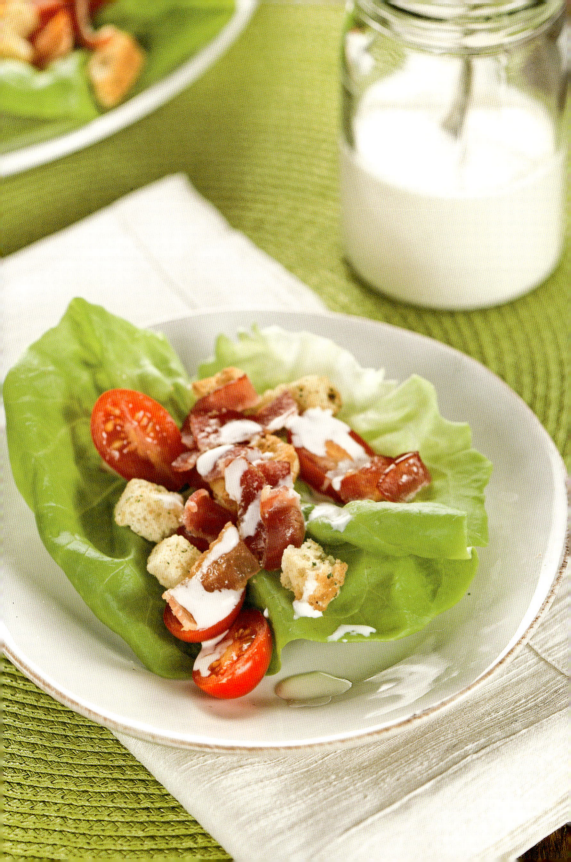

CROSTINI

Makes 16 appetizers (2 crostinis per serving)

1 whole wheat mini baguette
(about 4 ounces)

4 plum tomatoes

1 cup (4 ounces) shredded
part-skim mozzarella cheese

3 tablespoons pesto sauce

1 Preheat oven to 400°F. Slice baguette into 16 very thin, diagonal slices. Slice each tomato lengthwise into four (¼-inch) slices.

2 Place baguette slices on ungreased baking sheet. Top each with 1 tablespoon cheese and 1 tomato slice.

3 Bake 8 minutes or until bread is lightly toasted and cheese is melted. Top each crostini with about ½ teaspoon pesto sauce. Serve warm.

Nutrition Information (per serving)

Calories 83, **Total Fat** 3g, **Saturated Fat** 2g, **Cholesterol** 9mg, **Sodium** 159mg, **Carbohydrates** 9g, **Dietary Fiber** 1g, **Protein** 5g

Dietary Exchanges: ½ Bread/Starch • ½ Meat • ½ Fat

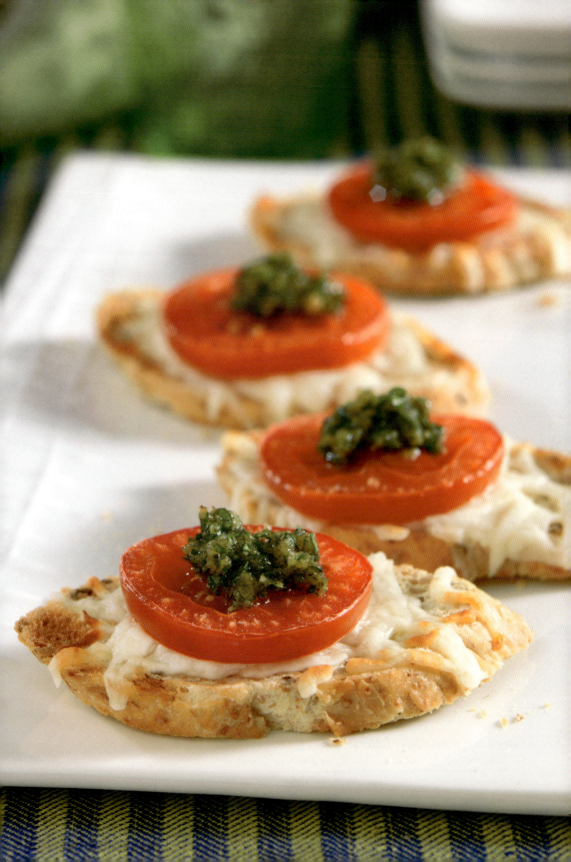

MINI SHRIMP SALAD ROLLS

Makes 12 servings (1 roll per serving)

¼ cup light mayonnaise

1 teaspoon chopped fresh dill

1 teaspoon fresh lemon juice

1 teaspoon hot pepper sauce

3 cups chopped cooked shrimp (about 1 pound)

1 package (12 ounces) sweet Hawaiian dinner rolls, split

6 lettuce leaves, torn in half

1 Stir mayonnaise, dill, lemon juice and hot pepper sauce in medium bowl until well blended. Add shrimp; gently mix to coat evenly.

2 To assemble, layer bottoms of rolls with lettuce, shrimp salad and tops of rolls.

Nutrition Information (per serving)

Calories 168, **Total Fat** 5g, **Saturated Fat** 2g, **Cholesterol** 98mg, **Sodium** 503mg, **Carbohydrates** 19g, **Dietary Fiber** 1g, **Protein** 13g

Dietary Exchanges: 1 Bread/Starch • 1 Meat

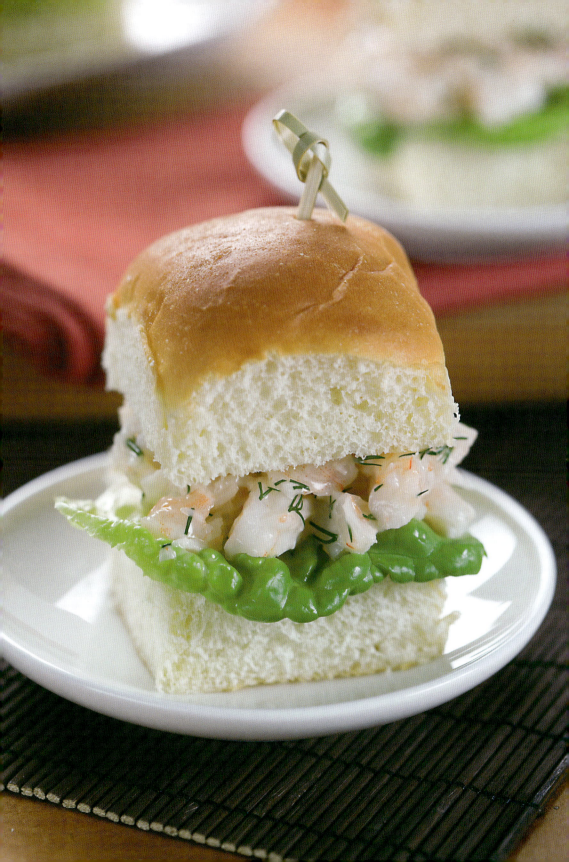

TURKEY & VEGGIE ROLL-UPS

Makes 2 servings (2 roll-ups per serving)

- 2 tablespoons hummus, any flavor
- 1 (8-inch) whole wheat tortilla
- ¼ cup sliced baby spinach
- 2 slices oven-roasted turkey breast (about 1 ounce)
- ¼ cup thinly sliced English cucumber
- 1 slice (1 ounce) reduced-fat Swiss cheese
- ¼ cup thinly sliced carrot

Spread hummus on tortilla to within 1 inch of edge. Layer with spinach, turkey, cucumber, cheese and carrots. Roll up tortilla and filling; cut into four pieces.

Nutrition Information (per serving)

Calories 140, **Total Fat** 4g, **Saturated Fat** 1g, **Cholesterol** 16mg, **Sodium** 292mg, **Carbohydrates** 14g, **Dietary Fiber** 2g, **Protein** 11g

Dietary Exchanges: 1 Bread/Starch • 1 Meat

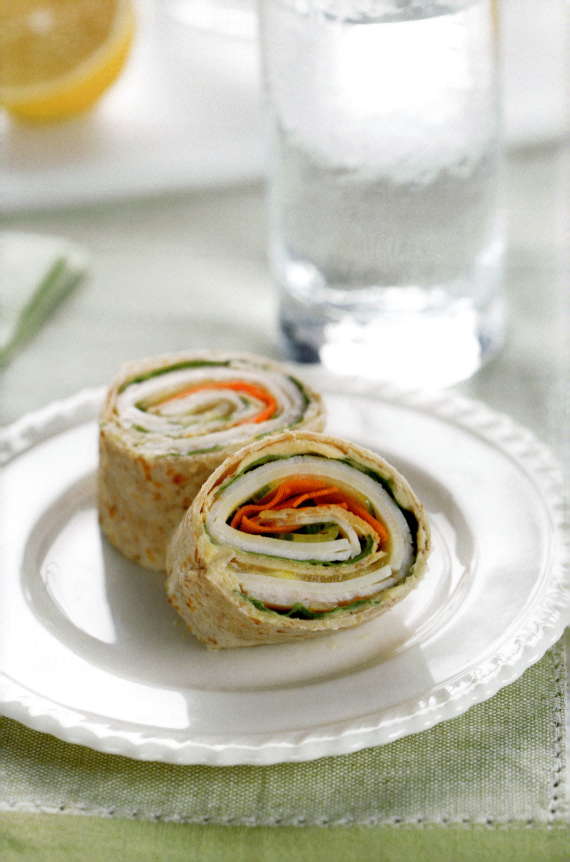

GREAT ZUKES PIZZA BITES

Makes 8 servings (2 pizza bites per serving)

1	medium zucchini
3	tablespoons pizza sauce
2	tablespoons tomato paste
¼	teaspoon dried oregano
¾	cup (3 ounces) shredded mozzarella cheese
¼	cup shredded Parmesan cheese
8	slices pitted black olives
8	slices pepperoni

1 Preheat broiler; set rack 4 inches from heat.

2 Trim off and discard ends of zucchini. Cut zucchini into 16 (¼-inch-thick) diagonal slices. Place on nonstick baking sheet.

3 Combine pizza sauce, tomato paste and oregano in small bowl; mix well. Spread scant teaspoon sauce over each zucchini slice. Combine cheeses in small bowl. Top each zucchini slice with 1 tablespoon cheese mixture, pressing down into sauce. Place 1 olive slice on each of 8 pizza bites. Place 1 folded pepperoni slice on each remaining pizza bite.

4 Broil 3 minutes or until cheese is melted. Serve immediately.

Nutrition Information (per serving)

Calories 75, **Total Fat** 5g, **Saturated Fat** 2g, **Cholesterol** 10mg, **Sodium** 288mg, **Carbohydrates** 3g, **Dietary Fiber** 1g, **Protein** 5g

Dietary Exchanges: ½ **Meat** • ½ **Vegetable**

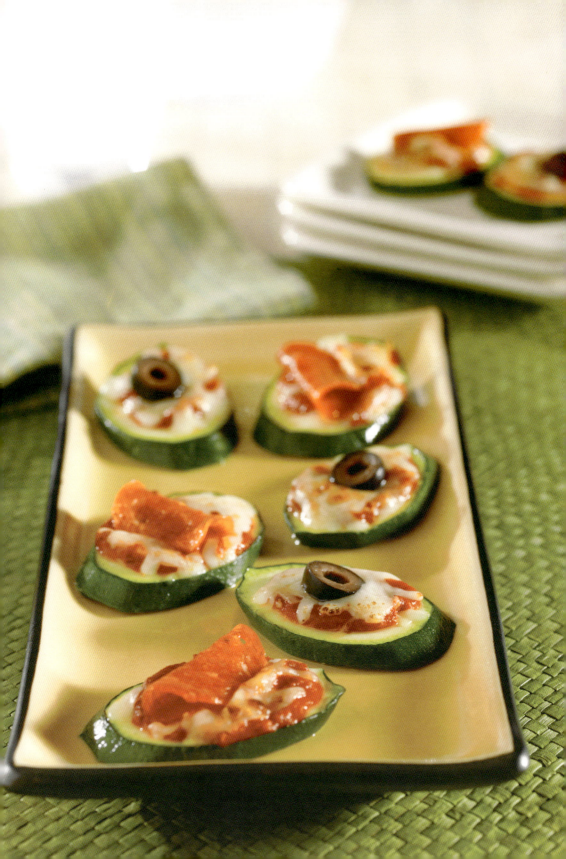

GARLIC-PARMESAN POPCORN

Makes 12 cups popcorn (2 cups per serving)

1 tablespoon olive oil

1 clove garlic, finely minced

1 tablespoon light butter-and-oil spread, melted

12 cups plain popped popcorn

⅓ cup finely grated Parmesan cheese

½ teaspoon dried basil

½ teaspoon dried oregano

Stir oil and garlic into spread in small bowl until well blended. Pour over popcorn in large bowl; toss to coat. Sprinkle with cheese, basil and oregano.

TIP: One regular-size microwavable package of popcorn yields about 10 to 12 cups of popped popcorn.

Nutrition Information (per serving)

Calories 110, **Total Fat** 5g, **Saturated Fat** 1g, **Cholesterol** 4mg, **Sodium** 83mg, **Carbohydrates** 13g, **Dietary Fiber** 2g, **Protein** 4g

Dietary Exchanges: 1 Bread/Starch • 1 Fat

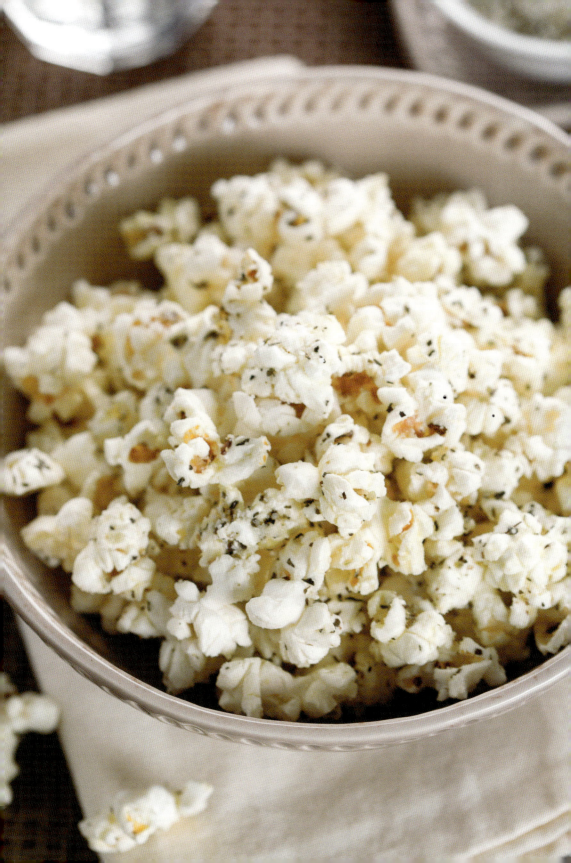

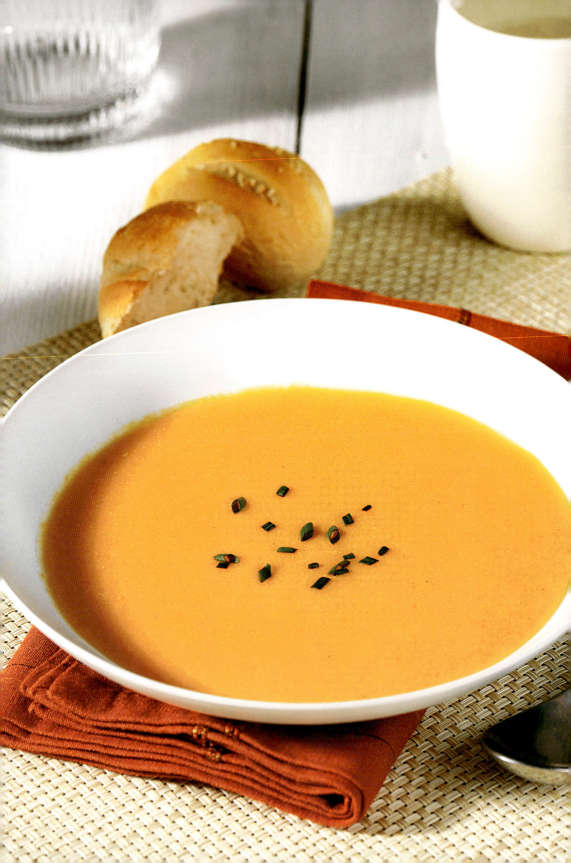

SOUPS & STEWS

SWEET POTATO BISQUE

Makes 4 servings

1 **pound sweet potatoes, peeled and cut into 2-inch chunks**

2 **teaspoons butter**

½ **cup finely chopped onion**

1 **teaspoon curry powder**

½ **teaspoon ground coriander**

¼ **teaspoon salt**

⅔ **cup unsweetened apple juice**

1 **cup buttermilk**

¼ **cup water (optional)**

Fresh snipped chives (optional)

Plain nonfat yogurt (optional)

1 Place sweet potatoes in large saucepan; cover with water. Bring to a boil over high heat. Cook 15 minutes or until potatoes are fork-tender. Drain; cool under cold running water.

2 Meanwhile, melt butter in small saucepan over medium heat. Add onion; cook and stir 2 minutes. Stir in curry powder, coriander and salt; cook and stir 1 minute or until onion is tender. Remove from heat; stir in apple juice.

3 Combine sweet potatoes, buttermilk and onion mixture in food processor or blender; cover and process until smooth. Return to saucepan; stir in ¼ cup water, if necessary, to thin to desired consistency. Cook and stir over medium heat until heated through. *Do not boil.* Garnish with chives or dollop of yogurt.

Nutrition Information (per serving)

Calories 160, **Total Fat** 3g, **Saturated Fat** 1g, **Cholesterol** 2mg, **Sodium** 231mg, **Carbohydrates** 31g, **Dietary Fiber** 4g, **Protein** 4g

Dietary Exchanges: 1½ **Bread/Starch** • ½ **Fruit** • ½ **Fat**

SAUSAGE VEGETABLE ROTINI SOUP

Makes 4 servings (1²/₃ cups per serving)

1	tablespoon olive oil
6	ounces bulk pork sausage
1	cup chopped onion
1	cup chopped green bell pepper
3	cups water
1	can (about 14 ounces) diced tomatoes
¼	cup ketchup
2	teaspoons beef bouillon granules
2	teaspoons chili powder
4	ounces uncooked tri-colored rotini pasta
1	cup frozen corn, thawed and drained

1 Heat oil in large saucepan over medium-high heat. Add sausage; cook 3 minutes or until no longer pink, stirring to break up sausage. Drain fat. Add onion and bell pepper; cook and stir 3 to 4 minutes or until onion is translucent.

2 Add water, tomatoes, ketchup, beef bouillon and chili powder; bring to a boil over high heat. Stir in pasta; return to a boil. Reduce heat to medium-low; simmer, uncovered, 12 minutes. Stir in corn; cook 2 minutes or until pasta is tender and corn is heated through.

Nutrition Information (per serving)

Calories 311, **Total Fat** 9g, **Saturated Fat** 2g, **Cholesterol** 31mg, **Sodium** 272mg, **Carbohydrates** 45g, **Dietary Fiber** 4g, **Protein** 14g

Dietary Exchanges: 2½ Bread/Starch • 1 Meat • ½ Vegetable • 1 Fat

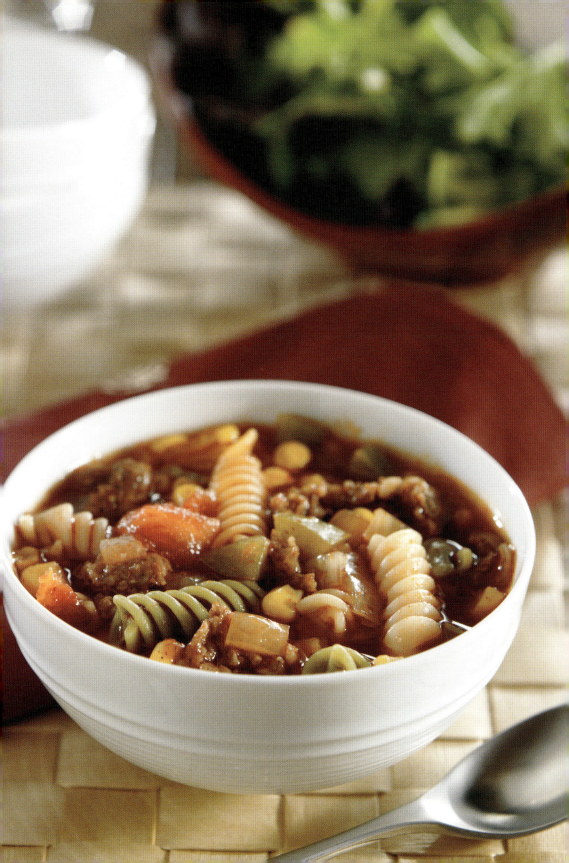

GROUND BEEF, SPINACH AND BARLEY SOUP

Makes 4 servings

12 ounces 95% lean ground beef

4 cups water

1 can (about 14 ounces) stewed tomatoes

1½ cups thinly sliced carrots

1 cup chopped onion

½ cup uncooked quick-cooking barley

1½ teaspoons beef bouillon granules

1½ teaspoons dried thyme

1 teaspoon dried oregano

½ teaspoon garlic powder

¼ teaspoon black pepper

⅛ teaspoon salt

3 cups fresh spinach leaves

1 Brown beef in large saucepan over medium-high heat 6 to 8 minutes, stirring to break up meat. Rinse beef under warm water; drain.

2 Return beef to saucepan; stir in 4 cups water, tomatoes, carrots, onion, barley, bouillon, thyme, oregano, garlic powder, pepper and salt; bring to a boil over high heat.

3 Reduce heat to medium-low. Cover; simmer 12 to 15 minutes or until barley and vegetables are tender, stirring occasionally. Stir in spinach; cook until spinach starts to wilt.

Nutrition Information (per serving)

Calories 265, **Total Fat** 6g, **Saturated Fat** 2g, **Cholesterol** 22mg, **Sodium** 512mg, **Carbohydrates** 33g, **Dietary Fiber** 8g, **Protein** 22g

Dietary Exchanges: 1 Bread/Starch • 2 Meat

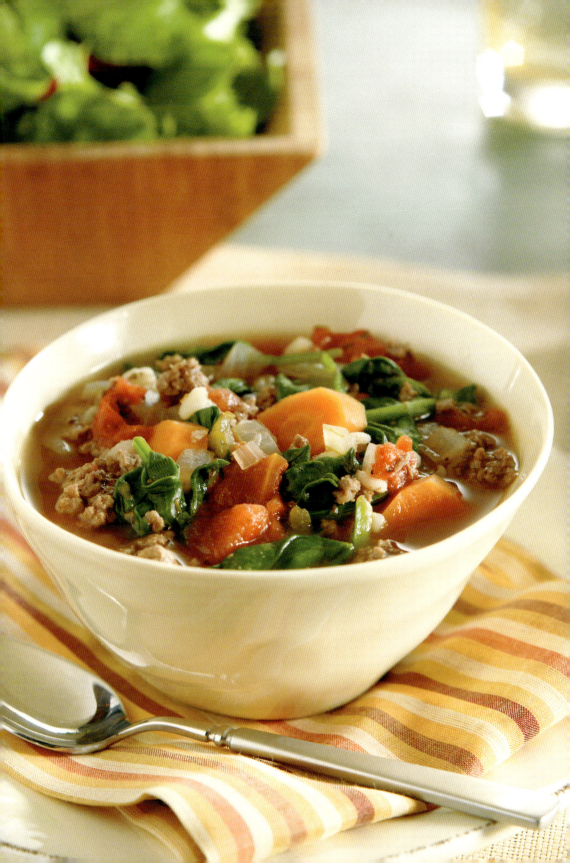

EGG DROP SOUP

Makes 2 servings (1½ cups per serving)

2 cans (about 14 ounces each) fat-free reduced-sodium chicken broth

1 tablespoon reduced-sodium soy sauce

2 teaspoons cornstarch

½ cup cholesterol-free egg substitute

¼ cup thinly sliced green onions

1 Bring broth to a boil in large saucepan over high heat. Reduce heat to medium-low.

2 Whisk soy sauce and cornstarch in small bowl until smooth and well blended; stir into broth. Cook and stir 2 minutes or until slightly thickened.

3 Stirring constantly in one direction, slowly pour egg substitute in thin stream into soup.

4 Ladle soup into bowls; sprinkle with green onions.

Nutrition Information (per serving)

Calories 45, **Total Fat** 1g, **Saturated Fat** 1g, **Cholesterol** 0mg, **Sodium** 243mg, **Carbohydrates** 3g, **Dietary Fiber** 1g, **Protein** 7g

Dietary Exchanges: 1 Meat

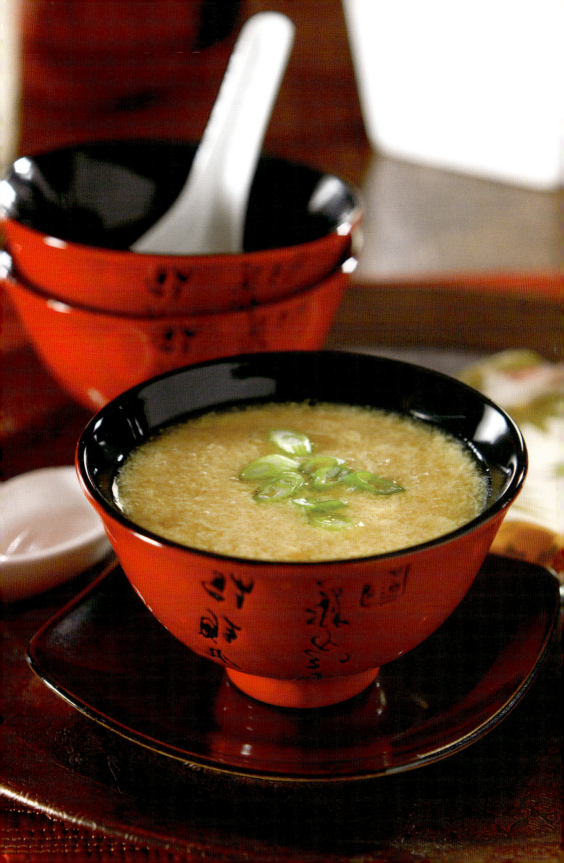

ITALIAN PASTA SOUP WITH FENNEL

Makes 6 servings (1 cup per serving)

1 tablespoon olive oil

1 small fennel bulb, trimmed and chopped into ¼-inch pieces (1½ cups)

4 cloves garlic, minced

3 cups vegetable broth

1 cup uncooked small shell pasta

1 medium zucchini or yellow summer squash, cut into ½-inch chunks

1 can (about 14 ounces) Italian-seasoned diced tomatoes

¼ cup grated Romano or Parmesan cheese

¼ cup chopped fresh basil

Dash black pepper (optional)

1 Heat oil in large saucepan over medium heat. Add fennel; cook and stir 5 minutes. Add garlic; cook and stir 30 seconds. Add broth and pasta; bring to a boil over high heat. Reduce heat; simmer 5 minutes. Stir in zucchini; simmer 5 to 7 minutes or until pasta and vegetables are tender.

2 Stir in tomatoes; heat through. Ladle into shallow bowls; top with cheese, basil and black pepper, if desired.

Nutrition Information (per serving)

Calories 126, **Total Fat** 4g, **Saturated Fat** 1g, **Cholesterol** 3mg, **Sodium** 430mg, **Carbohydrates** 17g, **Dietary Fiber** 2g, **Protein** 5g

Dietary Exchanges: 1 Bread/Starch • 1 Fat

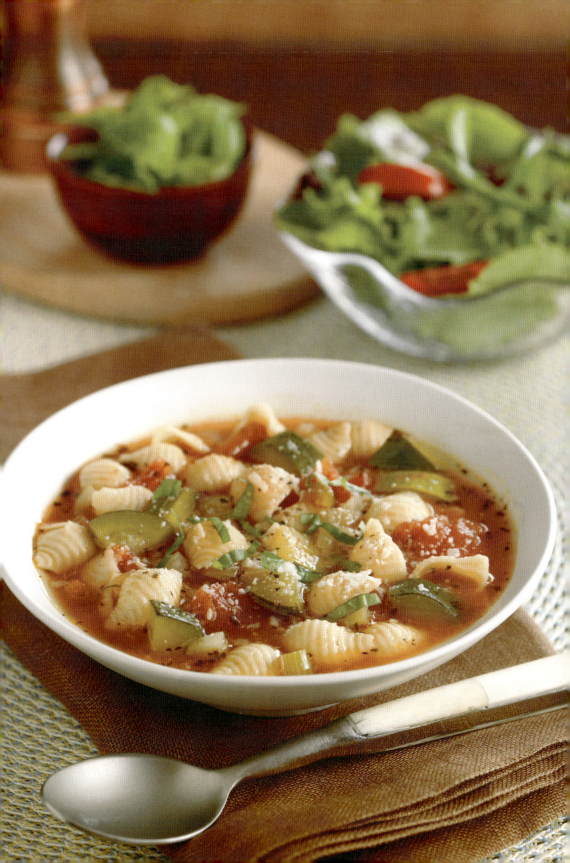

SLOW COOKER VEGGIE STEW

Makes 4 to 6 servings

1 tablespoon vegetable oil

⅔ cup carrot slices

½ cup diced onion

2 cloves garlic, chopped

2 cans (about 14 ounces each) vegetable broth

1½ cups chopped green cabbage

½ cup cut green beans

½ cup diced zucchini

1 tablespoon tomato paste

½ teaspoon dried basil

½ teaspoon dried oregano

¼ teaspoon salt

SLOW COOKER DIRECTIONS

1 Heat oil in medium skillet over medium-high heat. Add carrot, onion and garlic; cook and stir until tender. Transfer to slow cooker.

2 Stir in remaining ingredients. Cover; cook on LOW 8 to 10 hours or on HIGH 4 to 5 hours.

Nutrition Information (per serving)

Calories 83, **Total Fat** 4g, **Saturated Fat** 1g, **Cholesterol** 0mg, **Sodium** 654mg, **Carbohydrates** 10g, **Dietary Fiber** 2g, **Protein** 3g

Dietary Exchanges: 2 Vegetable • 1 Fat

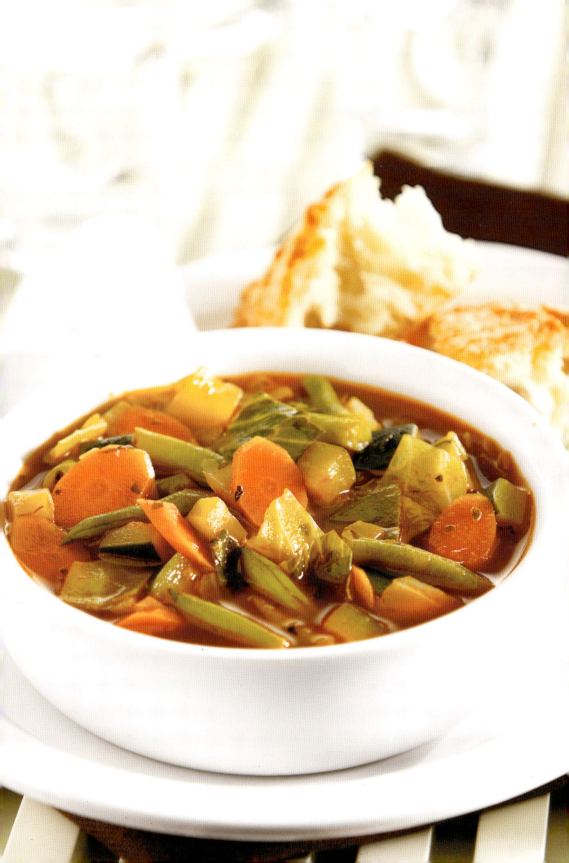

SKILLET CHICKEN SOUP

Makes 6 servings

¾ pound boneless skinless chicken breasts or thighs, cut into ¾-inch pieces

1 teaspoon paprika

½ teaspoon salt

¼ teaspoon black pepper

2 teaspoons vegetable oil

1 large onion, chopped

1 red bell pepper, cut into ½-inch pieces

3 cloves garlic, minced

3 cups fat-free reduced-sodium chicken broth

1 can (19 ounces) reduced-sodium cannellini beans or small white beans, rinsed and drained

3 cups sliced savoy or napa cabbage

½ cup fat-free herb-flavored croutons, slightly crushed (optional)

1 Toss chicken with paprika, salt and black pepper in medium bowl until coated.

2 Heat oil in large, deep nonstick skillet over medium-high heat until hot. Add chicken, onion, bell pepper and garlic. Cook until chicken is cooked through, stirring frequently.

3 Add broth and beans; bring to a simmer. Cover and simmer 5 minutes. Stir in cabbage; cover and simmer 3 additional minutes or until cabbage is wilted. Ladle into six shallow bowls; top evenly with crushed croutons, if desired.

TIP: Savoy cabbage, also called curly cabbage, is round with pale green crinkled leaves. Napa cabbage is also known as Chinese cabbage and is elongated with light green stalks.

Nutrition Information (per serving)

Calories 190, **Total Fat** 3.5g, **Saturated Fat** 0.5g, **Cholesterol** 40mg, **Sodium** 590mg, **Carbohydrates** 21g, **Dietary Fiber** 6g, **Protein** 19g

Dietary Exchanges: 1 Bread/Starch • 2 Meat • 1 Vegetable

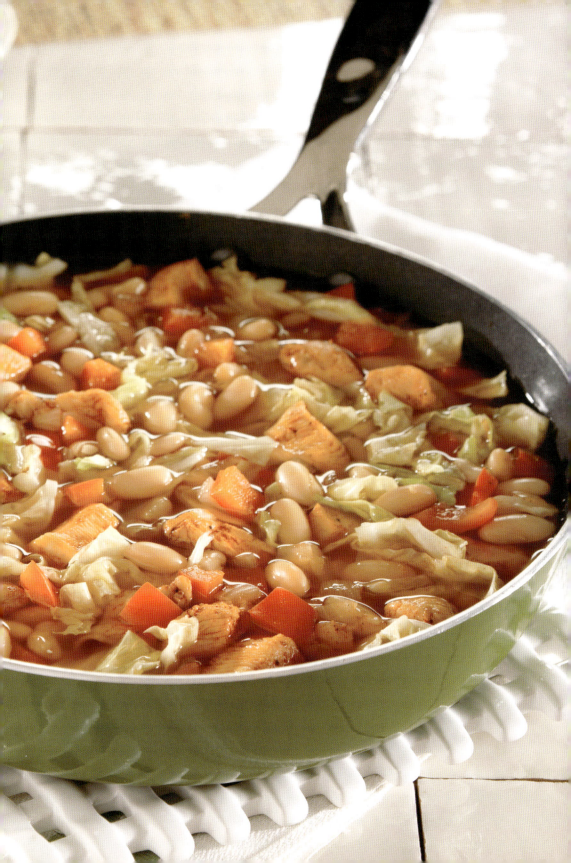

SWEET POTATO MINESTRONE

Makes 4 servings (1½ cups per serving)

1 tablespoon extra virgin olive oil

¾ cup diced onion

½ cup diced celery

3 cups water

2 cups diced peeled sweet potatoes

1 can (about 15 ounces) Great Northern beans, rinsed and drained

1 can (about 14 ounces) no-salt-added diced tomatoes

¾ teaspoon dried rosemary

½ teaspoon salt (optional)

⅛ teaspoon black pepper

2 cups coarsely chopped kale leaves (lightly packed)

4 tablespoons grated Parmesan cheese

1 Heat oil in large saucepan or Dutch oven over medium-high heat. Add onion and celery; cook and stir 4 minutes or until onion is softened. Stir water, sweet potatoes, beans, tomatoes, rosemary, salt, if desired, and pepper into saucepan. Cover and bring to a simmer; reduce heat and simmer 30 minutes.

2 Add kale; cover and cook 10 minutes or until tender.

3 Ladle soup into bowls; sprinkle with cheese.

NOTE: Choose kale in small bunches with firm leaves and a rich, deep color. Avoid bunches with limp, wilted or discolored leaves. To remove the tough stems, make a "V-shaped" cut where the stem joins the leaf. Stack the leaves and cut them into pieces.

Nutrition Information (per serving)

Calories 286, **Total Fat** 6g, **Saturated Fat** 2g, **Cholesterol** 4mg, **Sodium** 189mg, **Carbohydrates** 48g, **Dietary Fiber** 11g, **Protein** 13g

Dietary Exchanges: 3 Bread/Starch • 1 Meat

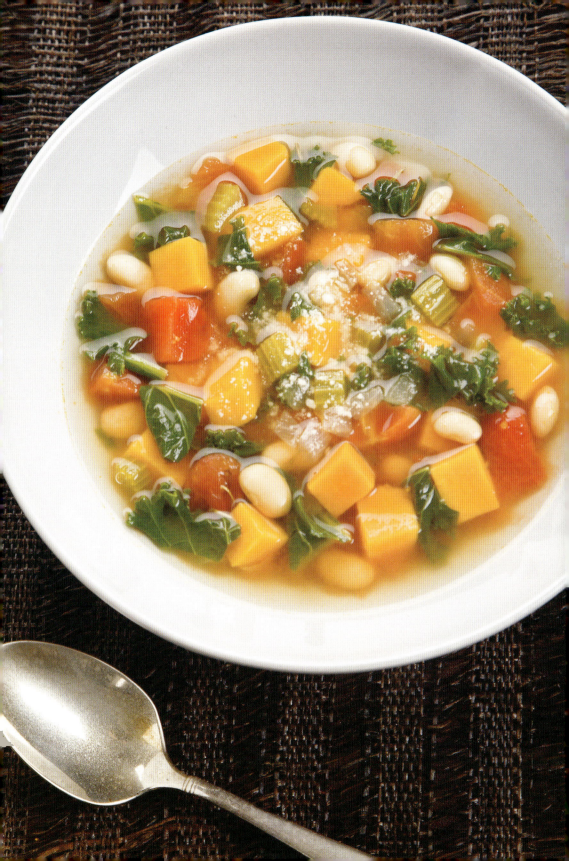

CHICKPEA-VEGETABLE SOUP

Makes 4 servings

1	teaspoon olive oil
1	cup chopped onion
½	cup chopped green bell pepper
2	cloves garlic, minced
2	cans (about 14 ounces each) no-salt-added chopped tomatoes
3	cups water
2	cups broccoli florets
1	can (about 15 ounces) chickpeas, rinsed, drained and slightly mashed
½	cup (3 ounces) uncooked orzo or rosamarina pasta
1	whole bay leaf
1	tablespoon chopped fresh thyme *or* 1 teaspoon dried thyme
1	tablespoon chopped fresh rosemary leaves *or* 1 teaspoon dried rosemary
1	tablespoon lime or lemon juice
½	teaspoon ground turmeric
¼	teaspoon salt
¼	teaspoon ground red pepper
¼	cup pumpkin seeds or sunflower kernels

1 Heat oil in large saucepan over medium heat. Add onion, bell pepper and garlic; cook and stir 5 minutes or until vegetables are tender.

2 Add tomatoes, water, broccoli, chickpeas, orzo, bay leaf, thyme, rosemary, lime juice, turmeric, salt and ground red pepper. Bring to a boil over high heat. Reduce heat to medium-low; cover and simmer 10 to 12 minutes or until orzo is tender.

3 Remove and discard bay leaf. Ladle soup into four serving bowls; sprinkle with pumpkin seeds.

Nutrition Information (per serving)

Calories 268, **Total Fat** 5g, **Saturated Fat** 1g, **Cholesterol** 0mg, **Sodium** 541mg, **Carbohydrates** 47g, **Dietary Fiber** 11g, **Protein** 12g

Dietary Exchanges: 2 Bread/Starch • 3 Vegetable • 1 Fat

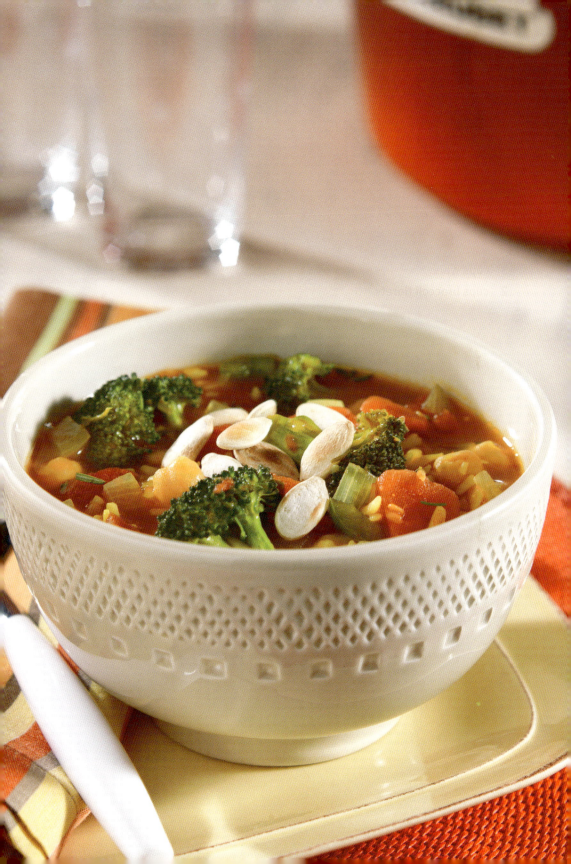

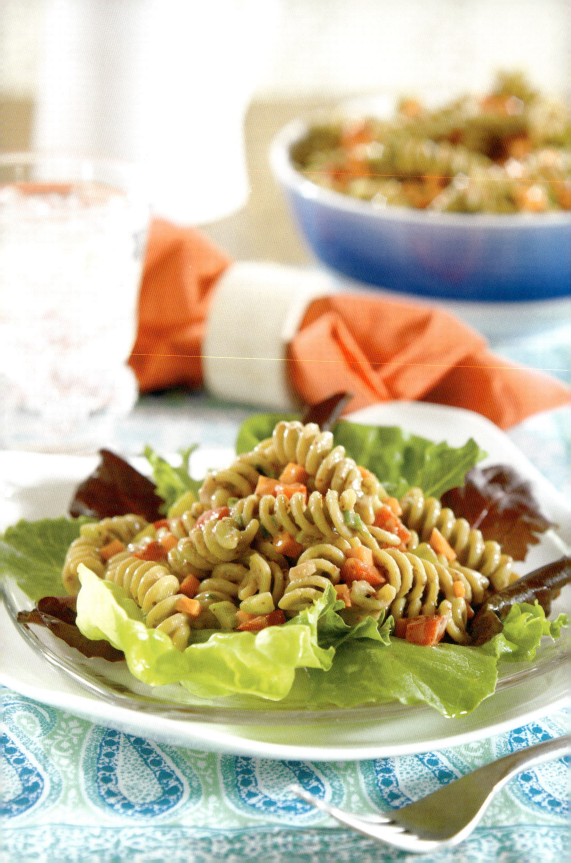

COLORFUL PASTA SALAD

Makes 8 servings

4 ounces uncooked spinach rotini or fusilli

⅓ cup finely chopped carrot

⅓ cup chopped celery

½ cup chopped red bell pepper

2 green onions with tops, sliced

3 tablespoons balsamic vinegar

2 tablespoons reduced-fat mayonnaise

2 teaspoons prepared whole grain mustard

½ teaspoon black pepper

¼ teaspoon Italian seasoning

Leaf lettuce

1 Cook pasta according to directions, omitting salt; drain. Rinse under cold running water until cool; drain.

2 Combine pasta, carrot, celery, bell pepper and green onions in medium bowl.

3 Whisk together vinegar, mayonnaise, mustard, black pepper and Italian seasoning in small bowl until blended. Pour over salad; toss to coat evenly. Cover and refrigerate up to 8 hours.

4 Arrange lettuce on individual plates. Spoon salad over lettuce.

Nutrition Information (per serving)

Calories 70, **Total Fat** 1g, **Saturated Fat** 0g, **Cholesterol** 0mg, **Sodium** 55mg, **Carbohydrates** 13g, **Dietary Fiber** 1g, **Protein** 2g

Dietary Exchanges: ½ Bread/Starch • ½ Vegetable

WARM CHUTNEY CHICKEN SALAD

Makes 2 servings

6 ounces boneless skinless chicken breasts, cut into bite-size pieces

⅓ cup mango chutney

¼ cup water

1 tablespoon Dijon mustard

4 cups packaged mixed salad greens

1 cup chopped peeled mango or papaya

Sliced green onions (optional)

1 Spray medium nonstick skillet with nonstick cooking spray. Heat over medium-high heat. Add chicken; cook and stir 2 to 3 minutes or until cooked through. Stir in chutney, water and mustard. Cook and stir just until hot. Cool slightly.

2 Toss together salad greens and mango in large bowl. Arrange on serving plates.

3 Spoon chicken mixture onto greens. Garnish with green onions.

Nutrition Information (per serving)

Calories 277, **Total Fat** 3g, **Saturated Fat** 1g, **Cholesterol** 52mg, **Sodium** 117mg, **Carbohydrates** 42g, **Dietary Fiber** 4g, **Protein** 21g

Dietary Exchanges: 2 Meat • 2 Fruit • 2 Vegetable

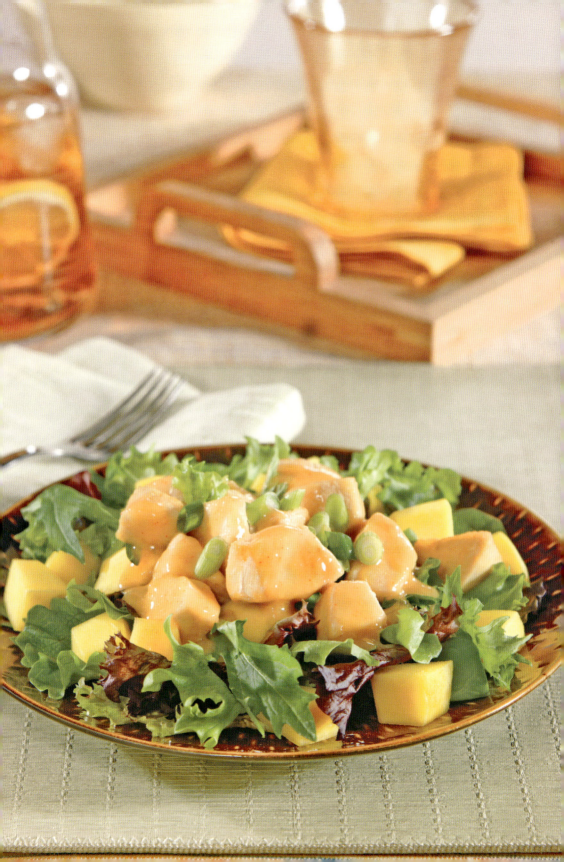

GRILLED SALMON SALAD WITH ORANGE-BASIL VINAIGRETTE

Makes 2 servings

¼ cup frozen orange juice concentrate, thawed

1 tablespoon plus 1½ teaspoons white wine vinegar or cider vinegar

1 tablespoon chopped fresh basil *or* 1 teaspoon dried basil

1½ teaspoons olive oil

1 salmon fillet (about 8 ounces and about 1 inch thick)

4 cups torn mixed greens

¾ cup sliced fresh strawberries

10 to 12 thin cucumber slices, cut into halves

⅛ teaspoon black pepper

1 Whisk orange juice concentrate, vinegar, basil and oil in small bowl until well blended. Remove 2 tablespoons orange juice mixture; reserve remaining mixture to use as salad dressing.

2 Prepare grill for direct cooking. Spray grid with nonstick cooking spray. Grill salmon, skin side down, over medium coals 5 minutes. Turn and grill 5 minutes or until fish flakes with fork, brushing frequently with 2 tablespoons juice concentrate mixture. Cool slightly.

3 Toss together greens, strawberries and cucumber in large bowl. Place on two serving plates.

4 Remove skin from salmon. Break salmon into chunks; arrange on greens mixture. Drizzle with reserved orange juice mixture; sprinkle with pepper.

Nutrition Information (per serving)

Calories 283, **Total Fat** 11g, **Saturated Fat** 2g, **Cholesterol** 60mg, **Sodium** 70mg, **Carbohydrates** 23g, **Dietary Fiber** 3g, **Protein** 24g

Dietary Exchanges: 3 Meat • 1½ Fruit • ½ Fat

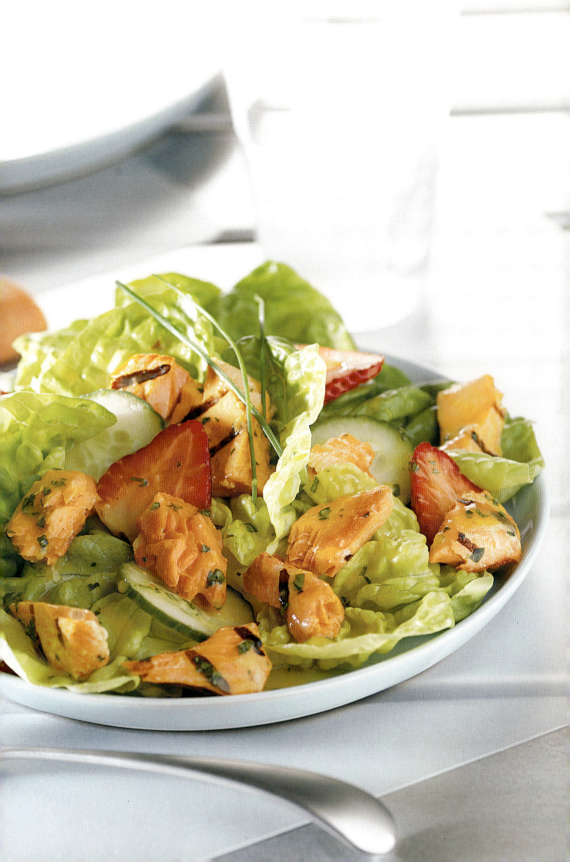

COUNTRY TIME MACARONI SALAD

Makes 6 servings (½ cup per serving)

½ cup (2 ounces) uncooked regular or whole wheat elbow macaroni

3 tablespoons reduced-fat mayonnaise

2 tablespoons plain nonfat yogurt

2 teaspoons sweet pickle relish

¾ teaspoon dried dill weed

½ teaspoon prepared yellow mustard (optional)

¼ teaspoon salt

½ cup frozen green peas

½ cup chopped green bell pepper

⅓ cup thinly sliced celery

4 ounces 99% fat-free ham, cubed

4 tablespoons (1 ounce) shredded reduced-fat Cheddar cheese, divided

1 Cook pasta according to package directions, omitting salt and fat; drain. Rinse under cold running water until completely cooled; drain.

2 Meanwhile, combine mayonnaise, yogurt, relish, dill weed, mustard, if desired, and salt in small bowl; stir until well blended.

3 Combine peas, bell pepper, celery and ham in medium bowl.

4 Add pasta and mayonnaise mixture to pea mixture; mix well. Stir in 2 tablespoons cheese; toss lightly. Sprinkle with remaining 2 tablespoons cheese. Serve immediately.

TIP: For best flavor, prepare the mayonnaise ingredients in a separate bowl at the time of serving.

Nutrition Information (per serving)

Calories 98, **Total Fat** 3g, **Saturated Fat** 1g, **Cholesterol** 12mg, **Sodium** 363mg, **Carbohydrates** 12g, **Dietary Fiber** 1g, **Protein** 7g

Dietary Exchanges: ½ Bread/Starch • ½ Meat • ½ Vegetable • ½ Fat

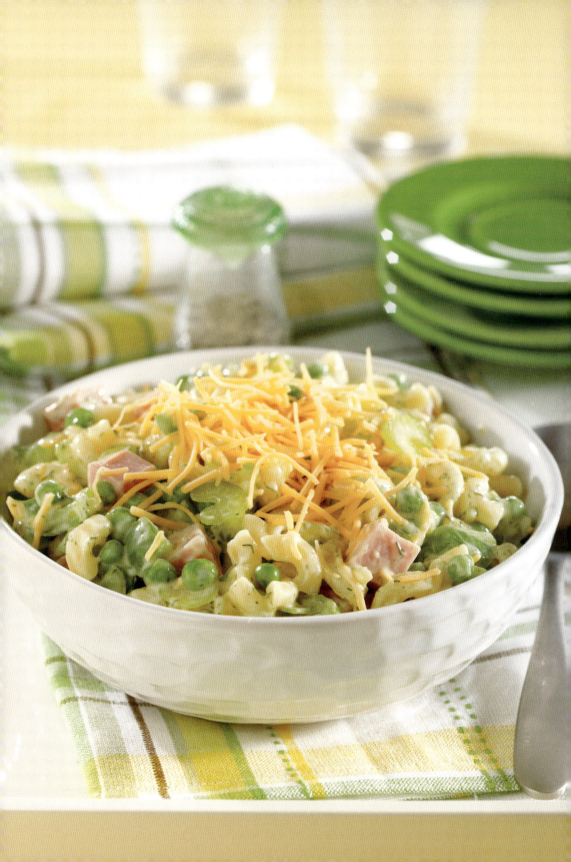

SPINACH-MELON SALAD

Makes 6 servings

6 cups packed fresh spinach

4 cups mixed melon balls (cantaloupe, honeydew and/ or watermelon)

1 cup zucchini ribbons*

½ cup sliced red bell pepper

¼ cup thinly sliced red onion

¼ cup red wine vinegar

2 tablespoons honey

2 teaspoons olive oil

2 teaspoons lime juice

1 teaspoon poppy seeds

1 teaspoon dried mint

To make ribbons, thinly slice zucchini lengthwise with vegetable peeler or spiral cutter.

1 Combine spinach, melon, zucchini, bell pepper and onion in large bowl.

2 Combine vinegar, honey, oil, lime juice, poppy seeds and mint in small jar with tight-fitting lid; shake well. Pour over salad; toss gently to coat.

Nutrition Information (per serving)

Calories 99, **Total Fat** 2g, **Saturated Fat** 1g, **Cholesterol** 0mg, **Sodium** 54mg, **Carbohydrates** 20g, **Dietary Fiber** 3g, **Protein** 3g

Dietary Exchanges: 1 Fruit • ½ Vegetable • ½ Fat

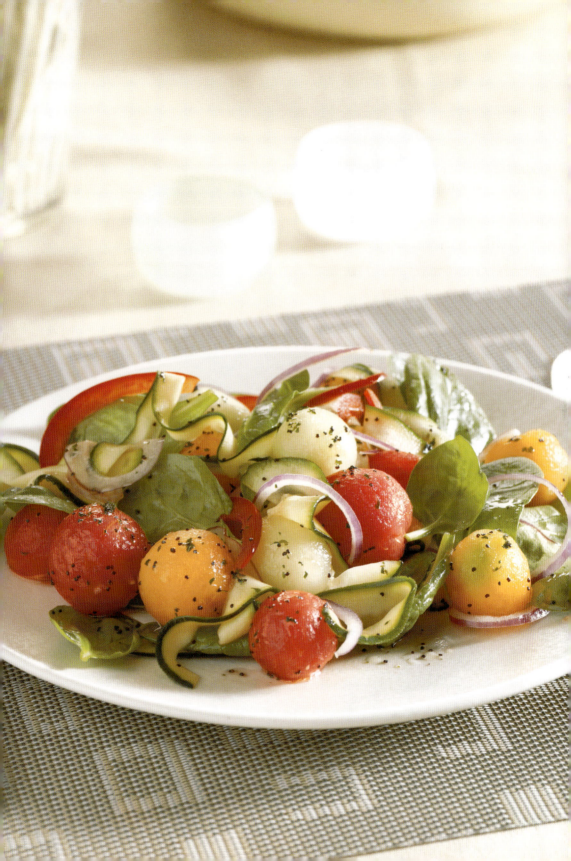

TOASTED PEANUT COUSCOUS SALAD

Makes 4 servings (½ cup per serving)

½   **cup water**

¼   **cup uncooked couscous**

1   **ounce unsalted dry-roasted peanuts**

½   **cup finely chopped red onion**

½   **cup finely chopped green bell pepper**

1   **tablespoon reduced-sodium soy sauce**

2   **teaspoons cider vinegar**

1½   **teaspoons sesame oil**

½   **teaspoon grated fresh ginger**

1   **packet sugar substitute**

¼   **teaspoon salt**

⅛   **teaspoon red pepper flakes**

1 Bring water to a boil in small saucepan over high heat. Remove from heat; stir in couscous. Cover tightly; let stand 5 minutes or until water is absorbed. Remove from pan to cool quickly, if desired.

2 Heat small nonstick skillet over medium-high heat until hot. Add peanuts; cook 2 to 3 minutes or until beginning to turn golden, stirring frequently.

3 Combine remaining ingredients in medium bowl. Add cooled couscous and toasted nuts; toss gently, yet thoroughly, to blend.

Nutrition Information (per serving)

Calories 115, **Total Fat** 5g, **Saturated Fat** 1g, **Cholesterol** 0mg, **Sodium** 298mg, **Carbohydrates** 14g, **Dietary Fiber** 2g, **Protein** 4g

Dietary Exchanges: 1 Bread/Starch · 1 Fat

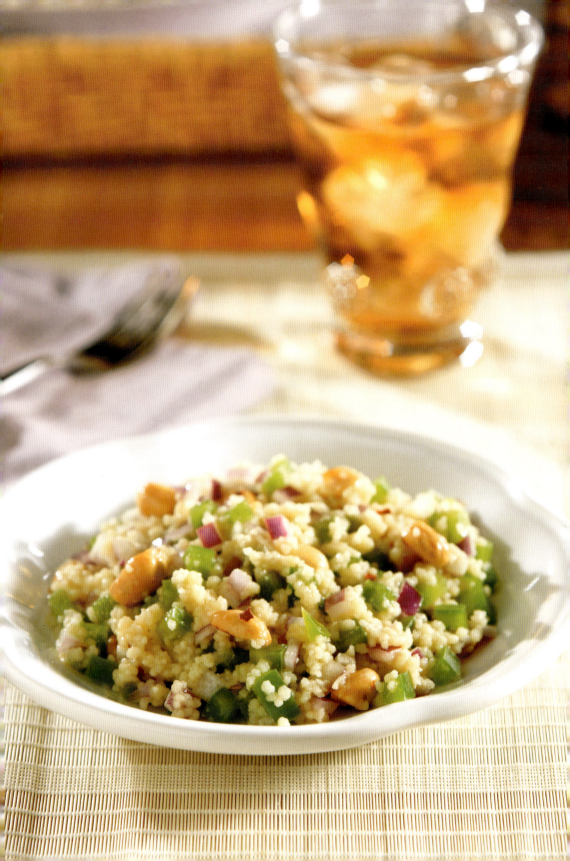

GARDEN POTATO SALAD WITH BASIL-YOGURT DRESSING

Makes 4 servings

3 cups water

6 new potatoes, quartered

8 ounces asparagus, cut into 1-inch slices

1¼ cups bell pepper strips

⅔ cup plain low-fat yogurt

¼ cup sliced green onions

2 tablespoons chopped pitted black olives

1½ tablespoons chopped fresh basil *or* 1½ teaspoons dried basil

1 tablespoon chopped fresh thyme *or* 1 teaspoon dried thyme

1 tablespoon white vinegar

2 teaspoons sugar

Dash ground red pepper

1 Bring 3 cups water to a boil in large saucepan over high heat. Add potatoes; return to a boil. Reduce heat to medium-low; cover and simmer 8 minutes. Add asparagus and bell peppers; cover and simmer 3 minutes or until potatoes are tender and asparagus and bell peppers are crisp-tender. Drain.

2 Meanwhile, combine yogurt, green onions, olives, basil, thyme, vinegar, sugar and ground red pepper in large bowl. Add vegetables; toss to coat. Cover and refrigerate at least 30 minutes or until chilled.

Nutrition Information (per serving)

Calories 154, **Total Fat** 3g, **Saturated Fat** 1g, **Cholesterol** 2mg, **Sodium** 173mg, **Carbohydrates** 30g, **Dietary Fiber** 3g, **Protein** 6g

Dietary Exchanges: 1½ Bread/Starch • 1 Vegetable • ½ Fat

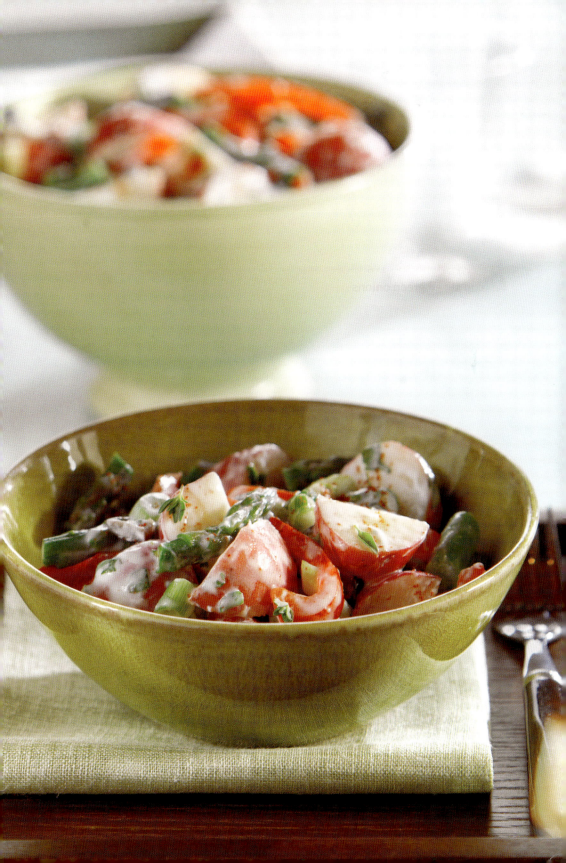

CARROT RAISIN SALAD WITH CITRUS DRESSING

Makes 8 servings

- ¾ cup light sour cream
- ¼ cup fat-free (skim) milk
- 1 tablespoon honey
- 1 tablespoon lime juice
- 1 tablespoon thawed frozen orange juice concentrate

  Grated peel of 1 medium orange
- ¼ teaspoon salt
- 8 medium carrots, peeled and coarsely shredded (about 2 cups)
- ¼ cup raisins
- ⅓ cup chopped cashew nuts

1 Stir sour cream, milk, honey, lime juice, orange juice concentrate, orange peel and salt in small bowl until smooth and well blended.

2 Combine carrots and raisins in large bowl. Add dressing; toss to coat. Cover and refrigerate 30 minutes. Gently toss before serving. Top with cashews.

Nutrition Information (per serving)

Calories 127, **Total Fat** 5g, **Saturated Fat** 2g, **Cholesterol** 8mg, **Sodium** 119mg, **Carbohydrates** 19g, **Dietary Fiber** 3g, **Protein** 4g

Dietary Exchanges: 1 Fruit • 1 Vegetable • 1 Fat

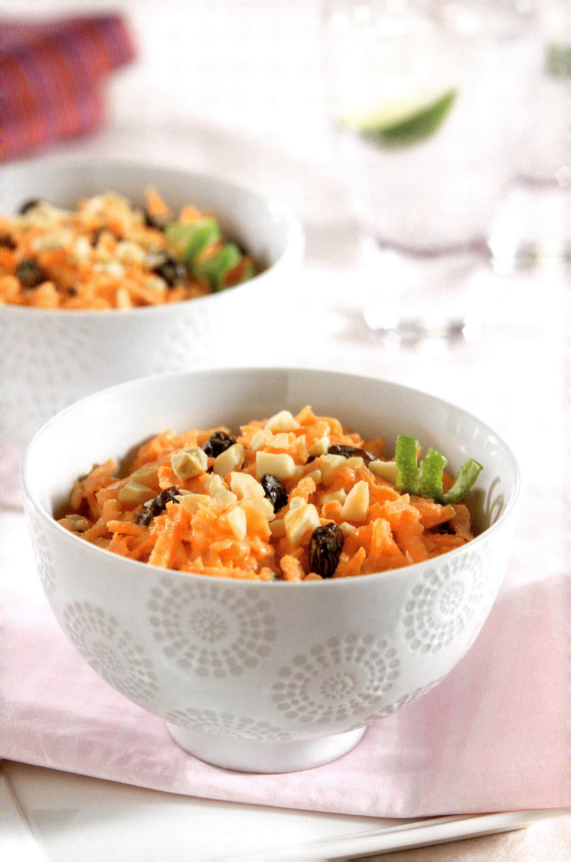

CRAB SPINACH SALAD WITH TARRAGON DRESSING

Makes 4 servings

12 ounces coarsely flaked cooked crabmeat *or* 2 packages (6 ounces each) frozen crabmeat, thawed and drained

1 cup chopped tomatoes

1 cup sliced cucumber

⅓ cup sliced red onion

¼ cup fat-free salad dressing or mayonnaise

¼ cup reduced-fat sour cream

¼ cup chopped fresh parsley

2 tablespoons fat-free (skim) milk

2 teaspoons chopped fresh tarragon *or* ½ teaspoon dried tarragon leaves

1 clove garlic, minced

¼ teaspoon hot pepper sauce

8 cups fresh spinach

1 Combine crabmeat, tomatoes, cucumber and onion in medium bowl. Combine salad dressing, sour cream, parsley, milk, tarragon, garlic and hot pepper sauce in small bowl.

2 Line four salad plates with spinach. Place crabmeat mixture on spinach; drizzle with dressing.

Nutrition Information (per serving)

Calories 170, **Total Fat** 4g, **Saturated Fat** 1g, **Cholesterol** 91mg, **Sodium** 481mg, **Carbohydrates** 14g, **Dietary Fiber** 4g, **Protein** 22g

Dietary Exchanges: 2½ **Meat** • 2 **Vegetable**

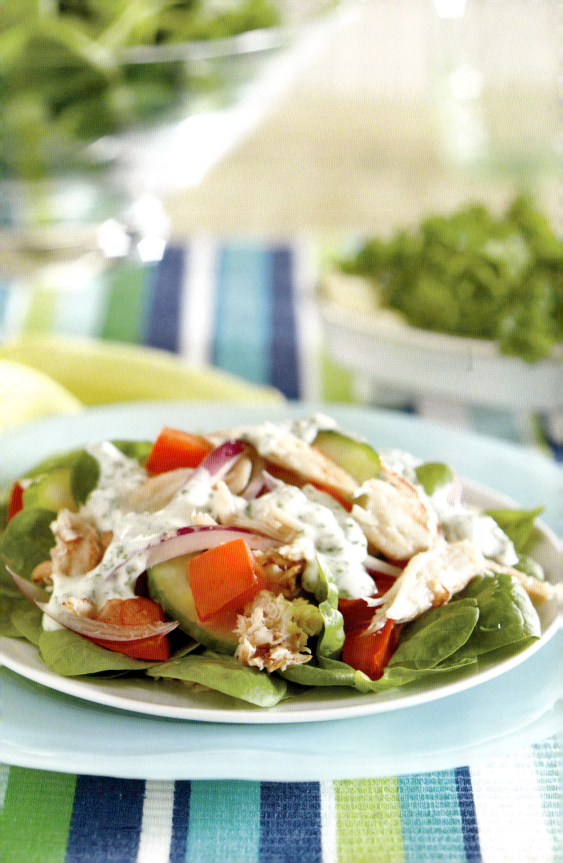

ARUGULA SALAD WITH SUN-DRIED TOMATO VINAIGRETTE

Makes 4 servings

¼ cup sun-dried tomatoes (not packed in oil)

2 tablespoons olive oil

1 tablespoon balsamic vinegar

¼ teaspoon salt

¼ teaspoon black pepper

1 package (5 ounces) baby arugula

1 cup halved grape tomatoes

¼ cup shaved Parmesan cheese

¼ cup pine nuts, toasted* (optional)

*To toast pine nuts, spread in single layer in heavy skillet. Cook over medium heat 1 to 2 minutes or until nuts are lightly browned, stirring frequently.

1 Combine sun-dried tomatoes, oil, vinegar, salt and pepper in blender or food processor; blend until smooth.

2 Combine arugula and grape tomatoes in large bowl. Add dressing; toss to coat. Top with cheese and pine nuts, if desired.

Nutrition Information (per serving)

Calories 114, **Total Fat** 9g, **Saturated Fat** 2g, **Cholesterol** 6mg, **Sodium** 274mg, **Carbohydrates** 6g, **Dietary Fiber** 1g, **Protein** 4g

Dietary Exchanges: 1 Vegetable • 2 Fat

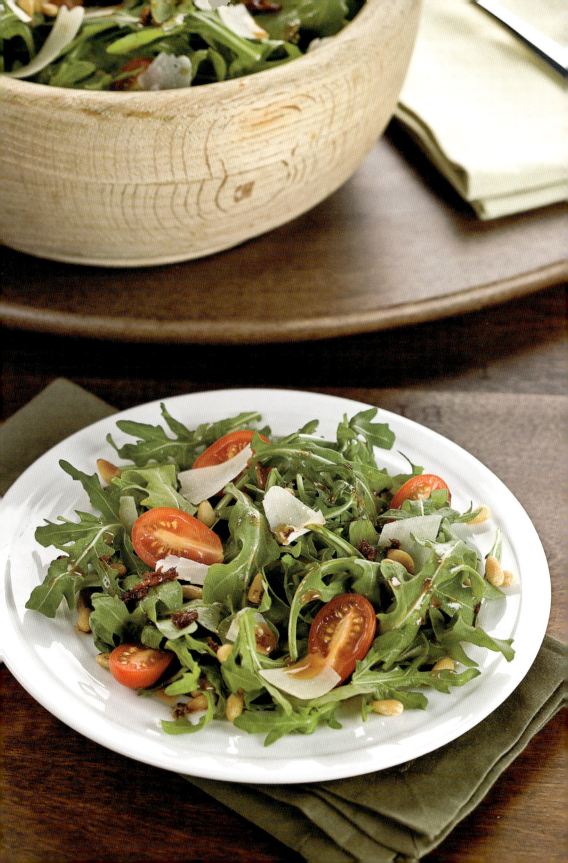

HEIRLOOM TOMATO QUINOA SALAD

Makes 4 servings (1 cup per serving)

1 cup uncooked quinoa

2 cups water

2 tablespoons olive oil

1 tablespoon lemon juice

1 clove garlic, minced

½ teaspoon salt

2 cups assorted heirloom grape tomatoes (red, yellow or a combination), halved

¼ cup crumbled fat-free feta cheese

¼ cup chopped fresh basil, plus additional basil leaves for garnish

1 Place quinoa in fine-mesh strainer; rinse well under cold running water. Bring 2 cups water to a boil in small saucepan; stir in quinoa. Reduce heat to low; cover and simmer 10 to 15 minutes or until quinoa is tender and water is absorbed.

2 Meanwhile, whisk oil, lemon juice, garlic and salt in large bowl until smooth and well blended. Gently stir in tomatoes and quinoa. Cover and refrigerate at least 30 minutes.

3 Stir in cheese just before serving. Top each serving with 1 tablespoon chopped basil. Garnish with additional basil leaves.

Nutrition Information (per serving)

Calories 246, **Total Fat** 10g, **Saturated Fat** 1g, **Cholesterol** 1mg, **Sodium** 387mg, **Carbohydrates** 32g, **Dietary Fiber** 4g, **Protein** 9g

Dietary Exchanges: 2 Bread/Starch • 1 Meat • 1 Fat

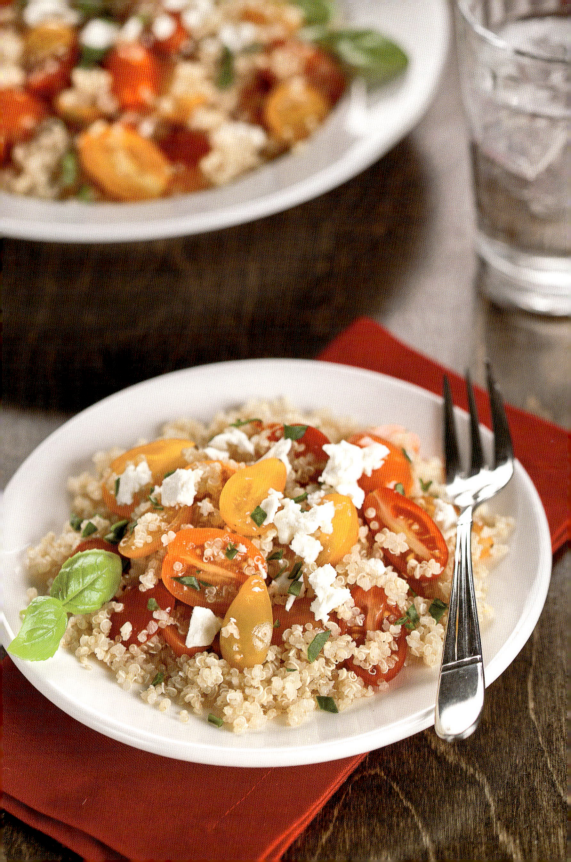

ZUCCHINI RIBBON SALAD

Makes 2 servings

2   medium zucchini

2   tablespoons chopped
    sun-dried tomatoes (not
    packed in oil)

2   teaspoons olive oil

1   teaspoon fresh lemon juice

1   teaspoon white vinegar

⅛   teaspoon salt

2   tablespoons shredded
    Parmesan cheese

1   tablespoon pine nuts, toasted*

To toast pine nuts, spread in single layer in heavy skillet. Cook over medium heat 1 to 2 minutes or until nuts are lightly browned, stirring frequently.

1 Cut zucchini into ribbons using vegetable peeler. Combine zucchini ribbons and sun-dried tomatoes in medium bowl.

2 Whisk oil, lemon juice, vinegar and salt in small bowl until well blended. Drizzle over zucchini and tomatoes; gently toss to coat.

3 Divide salad evenly between two serving bowls. Top with cheese and pine nuts. Serve immediately.

Nutrition Information (per serving)

Calories 133, **Total Fat** 10g, **Saturated Fat** 2g, **Cholesterol** 4mg, **Sodium** 254mg, **Carbohydrates** 9g, **Dietary Fiber** 3g, **Protein** 5g

Dietary Exchanges: 2 Vegetable • 2 Fat

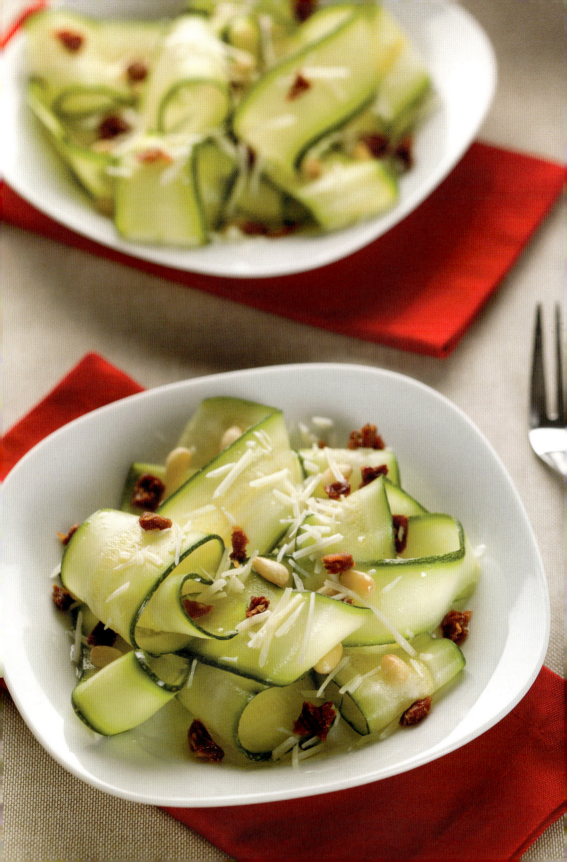

ROASTED SWEET POTATO AND APPLE SALAD

Makes 4 servings

2 large sweet potatoes, peeled and cubed

½ teaspoon salt, divided

¼ teaspoon black pepper

3 tablespoons low-calorie apple juice cocktail

1 tablespoon olive oil

1 tablespoon balsamic vinegar

1 tablespoon Dijon mustard

1 tablespoon honey

2 teaspoons snipped fresh chives

1 medium Gala apple, diced (about 1 cup)

½ cup finely chopped celery

¼ cup thinly sliced red onion

Lettuce leaves

1 Preheat oven to 450°F. Arrange sweet potatoes in single layer on baking sheet. Spray with nonstick cooking spray; season with ¼ teaspoon salt and pepper.

2 Roast 20 to 25 minutes or until potatoes are tender, stirring halfway through cooking time. Cool completely.

3 Meanwhile, whisk apple juice cocktail, oil, vinegar, mustard, honey, chives and remaining ¼ teaspoon salt in small bowl until smooth and well blended.

4 Combine sweet potatoes, apple, celery and onion in medium bowl. Drizzle with dressing; gently toss to coat. Arrange lettuce leaves on four serving plates. Top evenly with sweet potato mixture.

Nutrition Information (per serving)

Calories 133, **Total Fat** 4g, **Saturated Fat** 1g, **Cholesterol** 0mg, **Sodium** 424mg, **Carbohydrates** 26g, **Dietary Fiber** 3g, **Protein** 1g

Dietary Exchanges: 1½ Bread/Starch • ½ Fat

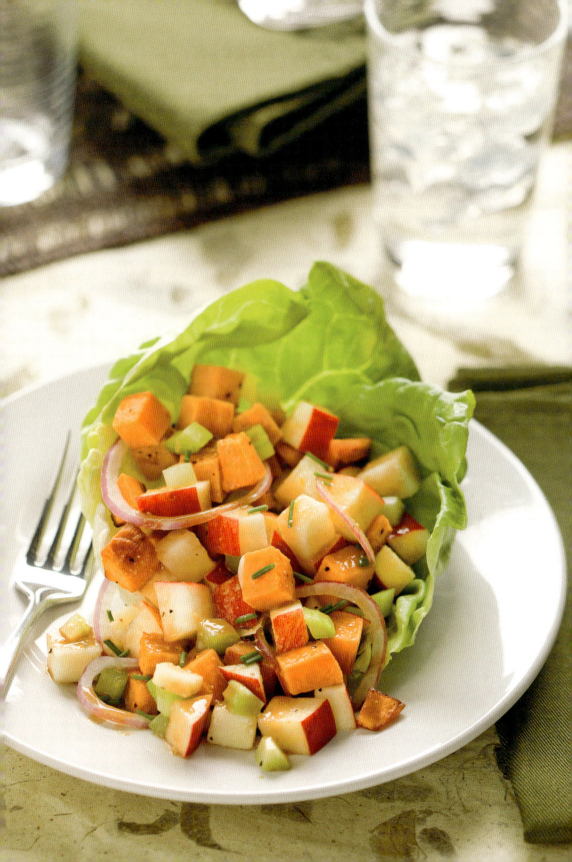

BROCCOLI SLAW WITH CHICKEN AND HONEY-LIME DRESSING

Makes 4 servings (2 cups salad and 2 tablespoons dressing per serving)

DRESSING

- ¼ **cup fresh lime juice**
- 1½ **tablespoons olive oil**
- 2 **tablespoons seasoned rice wine vinegar**
- 2 **teaspoons honey**
- 1 **teaspoon ground cumin**
- 1 **small clove garlic, crushed**
- ¼ **teaspoon salt**
- ¼ **teaspoon black pepper**

SLAW

- 2 **bags (9 ounces each) broccoli coleslaw**
- 2 **cups shredded cooked chicken**
- 1 **cup black beans, rinsed and drained**
- ½ **cup thinly sliced green onions**

1 Combine dressing ingredients in small bowl; whisk until well combined. Set aside.

2 Place broccoli coleslaw and remaining ingredients in large bowl; toss gently to combine.

3 Drizzle dressing over slaw; toss gently to coat. Refrigerate at least 1 hour to let flavors blend. Toss before serving.

Nutrition Information (per serving)

Calories 272, **Total Fat** 10g, **Saturated Fat** 2g, **Cholesterol** 58mg, **Sodium** 555mg, **Carbohydrates** 24g, **Dietary Fiber** 7g, **Protein** 26g

Dietary Exchanges: 1 Bread/Starch • 3 Meat • 1 Vegetable

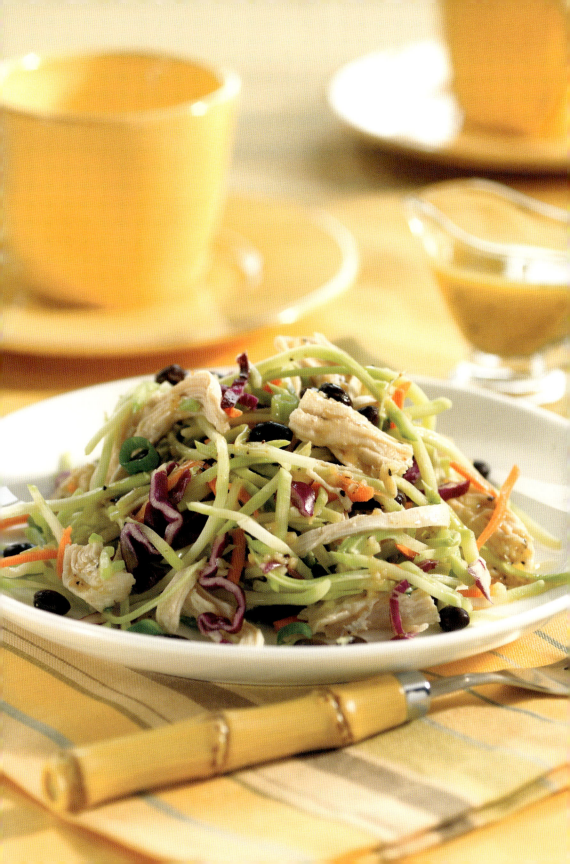

CRAB AND PASTA SALAD IN CANTALOUPE

Makes 4 servings

1½	cups uncooked rotini pasta
1	cup seedless green grapes
½	cup chopped celery
½	cup fresh pineapple chunks
1	small red onion, coarsely chopped
6	ounces canned, fresh or frozen crabmeat, drained
½	cup plain nonfat yogurt
¼	cup light mayonnaise
2	tablespoons fresh lemon juice
2	tablespoons honey
2	teaspoons grated lemon peel
1	teaspoon Dijon mustard
2	small cantaloupes

1 Cook rotini according to package instructions, omitting salt; drain. Rinse under cold running water; drain. Set aside.

2 Combine grapes, celery, pineapple, onion and crabmeat in large bowl. Combine yogurt, mayonnaise, lemon juice, honey, lemon peel and mustard in small bowl. Add yogurt mixture and reserved pasta to crabmeat mixture. Toss to coat evenly. Cover and refrigerate.

3 Just before serving, cut cantaloupes in half. Remove and discard seeds. Remove some of cantaloupe with spoon, leaving a shell about ¾ inch thick. Fill cantaloupe with salad.

Nutrition Information (per serving)

Calories 331, **Total Fat** 6g, **Saturated Fat** 1g, **Cholesterol** 42mg, **Sodium** 463mg, **Carbohydrates** 56g, **Dietary Fiber** 1g, **Protein** 14g

Dietary Exchanges: 1½ Bread/Starch • 1½ Meat • 1½ Fruit • ½ Vegetable • 1 Fat

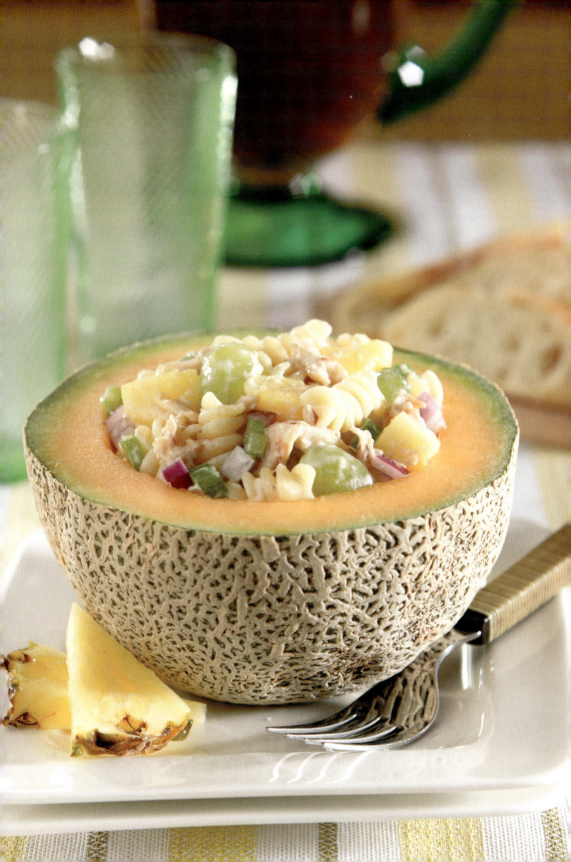

MARINATED BEAN AND VEGETABLE SALAD

Makes 8 servings (½ cup per serving)

¼ cup orange juice

3 tablespoons white wine vinegar

1 tablespoon canola or vegetable oil

2 cloves garlic, minced

1 can (about 15 ounces) Great Northern beans, rinsed and drained

1 can (about 15 ounces) kidney beans, rinsed and drained

¼ cup coarsely chopped red cabbage

¼ cup chopped red onion

¼ cup chopped green bell pepper

¼ cup chopped red bell pepper

¼ cup sliced celery

1 Combine orange juice, vinegar, oil and garlic in small jar with tight-fitting lid; shake well.

2 Combine beans, cabbage, onion, bell peppers and celery in large bowl. Pour dressing over bean mixture; toss to coat.

3 Refrigerate, covered, 1 to 2 hours to allow flavors to blend. Toss before serving.

Nutrition Information (per serving)

Calories 136, **Total Fat** 2g, **Saturated Fat** 1g, **Cholesterol** 0mg, **Sodium** 180mg, **Carbohydrates** 23g, **Dietary Fiber** 3g, **Protein** 7g

Dietary Exchanges: 1 Bread/Starch • 1½ Vegetable • ½ Fat

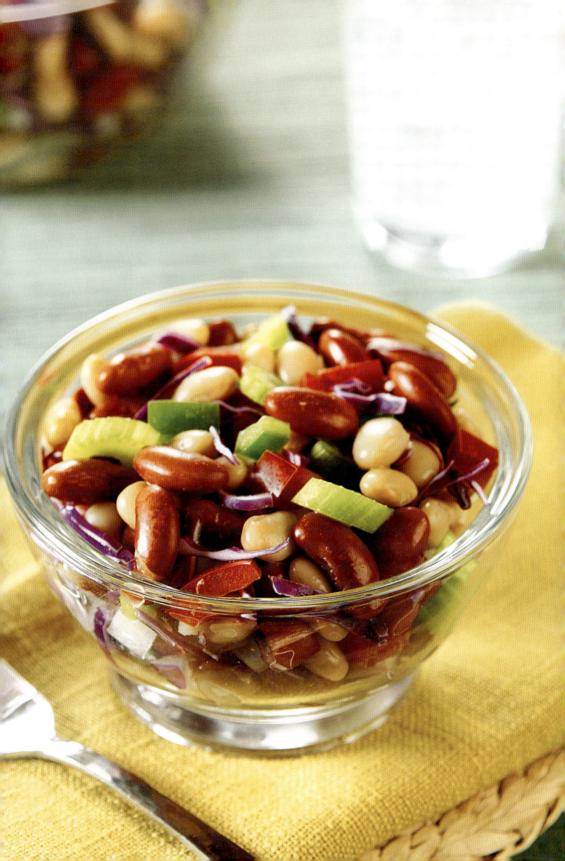

SPINACH SALAD WITH POMEGRANATE VINAIGRETTE

Makes 4 servings

1   package (5 ounces) baby spinach

½   cup pomegranate seeds (arils)

¼   cup crumbled goat cheese

2   tablespoons chopped walnuts, toasted*

¼   cup pomegranate juice

2   tablespoons olive oil

1   tablespoon red wine vinegar

1   tablespoon honey

¼   teaspoon salt

¼   teaspoon black pepper

*To toast walnuts, spread in single layer in heavy-bottomed skillet. Cook over medium heat 1 to 2 minutes, stirring frequently, until nuts are lightly browned. Remove from skillet immediately. Cool before using.

1 Combine spinach, pomegranate seeds, goat cheese and walnuts in large bowl.

2 Whisk pomegranate juice, oil, vinegar, honey, salt and pepper in small bowl until well blended. Pour over salad; gently toss to coat. Serve immediately.

TIP: For easier removal of pomegranate seeds, cut a pomegranate into pieces and immerse in a bowl of cold water. The membrane that holds the seeds in place will float to the top; discard it and collect the seeds. For convenience, you can find containers of ready-to-use pomegranate seeds in the refrigerated produce section of some supermarkets.

Nutrition Information (per serving)

Calories 161, **Total Fat** 11g, **Saturated Fat** 3g, **Cholesterol** 4mg, **Sodium** 210mg, **Carbohydrates** 12g, **Dietary Fiber** 1g, **Protein** 4g

Dietary Exchanges: 2 Vegetable • 2½ Fat

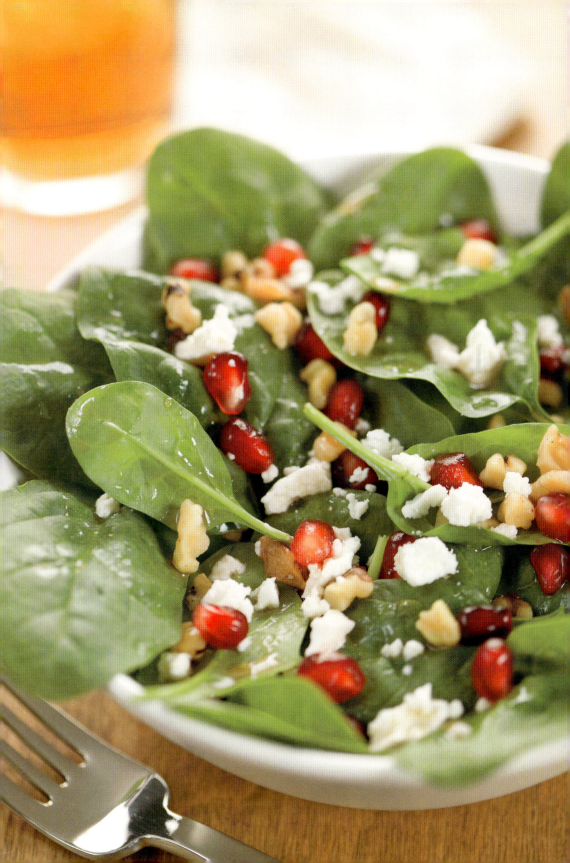

SWEET & SAVORY SWEET POTATO SALAD

Makes 6 servings (¾ cup per serving)

4 cups peeled chopped cooked sweet potatoes (about 4 to 6)

¾ cup chopped green onions

½ cup chopped fresh parsley

½ cup dried unsweetened cherries

¼ cup plus 2 tablespoons rice wine vinegar

2 tablespoons coarse ground mustard

1 tablespoon extra virgin olive oil

¾ teaspoon garlic powder

¼ teaspoon black pepper

⅛ teaspoon salt

1 Combine sweet potatoes, green onions, parsley and cherries in large bowl; gently mix.

2 Whisk vinegar, mustard, oil, garlic powder, pepper and salt in small bowl until well blended. Pour over sweet potato mixture; gently toss to coat. Serve immediately or cover and refrigerate until ready to serve.

Nutrition Information (per serving)

Calories 161, **Total Fat** 3g, **Saturated Fat** 0g, **Cholesterol** 0mg, **Sodium** 116mg, **Carbohydrates** 33g, **Dietary Fiber** 4g, **Protein** 3g

Dietary Exchanges: 2 Bread/Starch • ½ Fat

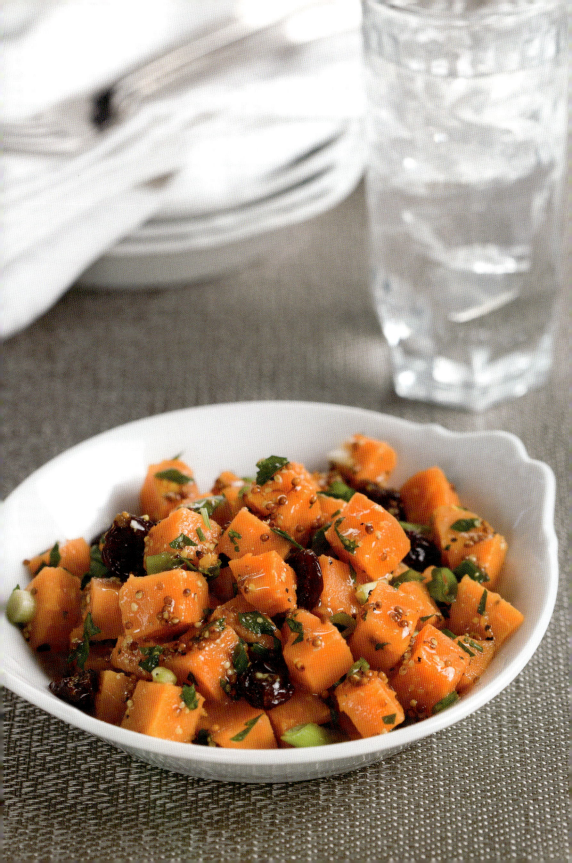

MANDARIN CHICKEN SALAD

Makes 4 servings

3½ ounces thin rice noodles (rice vermicelli)

1 can (6 ounces) mandarin orange segments, chilled

⅓ cup honey

2 tablespoons rice wine vinegar

2 tablespoons reduced-sodium soy sauce

1 can (8 ounces) sliced water chestnuts, drained

4 cups shredded napa cabbage

1 cup shredded red cabbage

½ cup sliced radishes

4 thin slices red onion, cut in half and separated

3 boneless skinless chicken breasts (about 12 ounces), cooked and cut into strips

1 Place rice noodles in large bowl. Cover with hot water; soak 20 minutes or until soft. Drain.

2 Drain mandarin orange segments, reserving ⅓ cup liquid. Whisk reserved liquid, honey, vinegar and soy sauce in medium bowl. Add water chestnuts.

3 Divide noodles, cabbages, radishes and onion evenly among four serving plates. Top with chicken and orange segments. Remove water chestnuts from dressing and arrange on salads. Serve with remaining dressing.

Nutrition Information (per serving)

Calories 258, **Total Fat** 2g, **Saturated Fat** 1g, **Cholesterol** 34mg, **Sodium** 318mg, **Carbohydrates** 46g, **Dietary Fiber** 2g, **Protein** 16g

Dietary Exchanges: 1 Bread/Starch • 2 Meat • ½ Fruit • 2 Vegetable

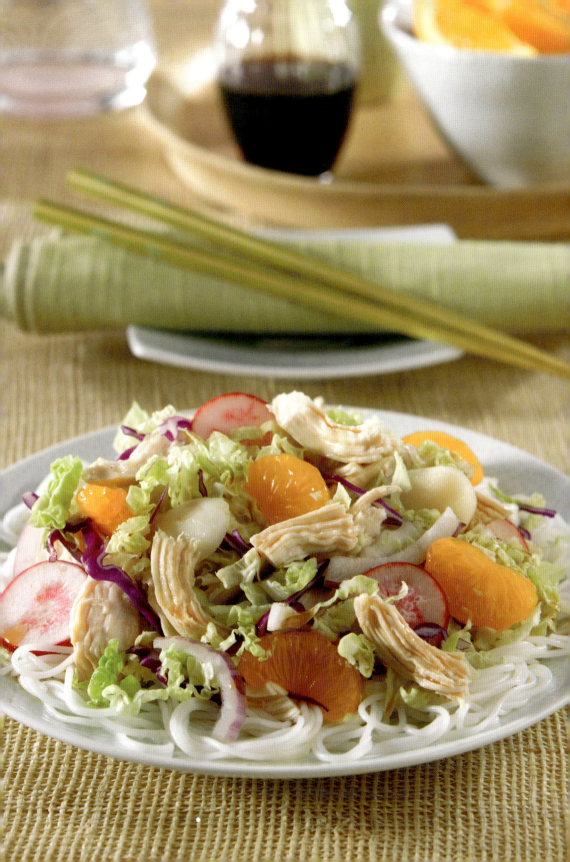

SWEET AND SOUR BROCCOLI PASTA SALAD

Makes 6 servings

8   ounces uncooked pasta twists

2   cups broccoli florets

⅔   cup shredded carrots

1   medium Red or Golden
    Delicious apple, cored,
    seeded and chopped

⅓   cup plain nonfat yogurt

⅓   cup apple juice

3   tablespoons cider vinegar

1   tablespoon olive oil

1   tablespoon Dijon mustard

1   teaspoon honey

½   teaspoon dried thyme

    Lettuce leaves

1 Cook pasta according to package directions, omitting salt; add broccoli during the last 2 minutes of cooking. Drain; rinse under cold running water until pasta and broccoli are cool. Drain.

2 Place pasta, broccoli, carrots and apple in medium bowl.

3 Stir yogurt, apple juice, vinegar, oil, mustard, honey and thyme in small bowl until smooth and well blended. Pour over pasta mixture; toss to coat.

4 Line six plates with lettuce. Top evenly with pasta salad. Garnish with apple slices, if desired.

Nutrition Information (per serving)

Calories 198, **Total Fat** 3g, **Saturated Fat** 1g, **Cholesterol** 1mg, **Sodium** 57mg, **Carbohydrates** 36g, **Dietary Fiber** 3g, **Protein** 7g

Dietary Exchanges: 2 Bread/Starch • ½ Fruit • ½ Vegetable • ½ Fat

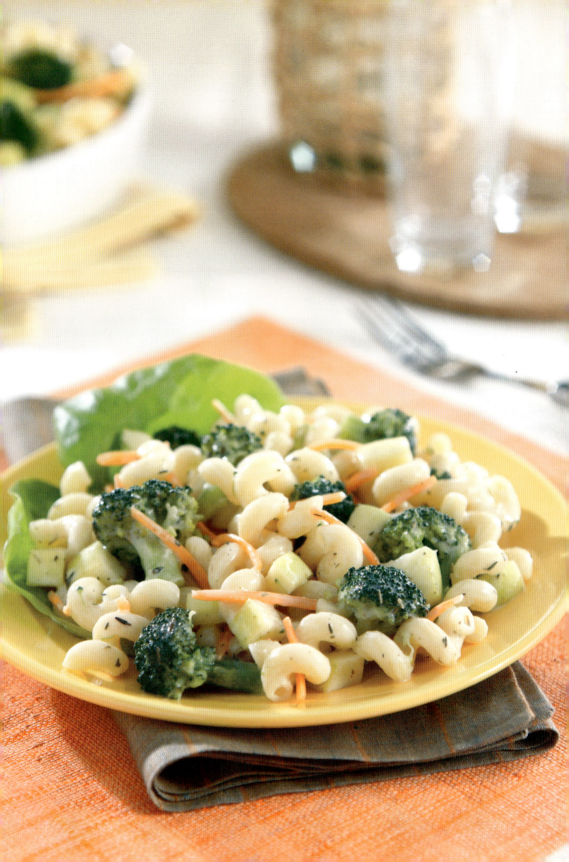

CHICKEN SATAY SALAD

Makes 4 servings

- ¼ cup plus 2 tablespoons peanut sauce, divided
- 2 tablespoons lime juice
- 1 tablespoon unseasoned rice vinegar
- 3 teaspoons toasted sesame oil, divided
- 1 pound chicken tenders, cut in half lengthwise
- 4 cups chopped romaine lettuce
- 1 red bell pepper, thinly sliced
- 1 cup shredded carrots
- 1 cup sliced Persian cucumbers*
- ¼ cup chopped fresh cilantro
- 1 tablespoon peanuts, chopped

Persian cucumbers are similar to English cucumbers; they have fewer seeds and contain less water than traditional cucumbers, which gives them a sweeter flavor and crunchier texture. These smaller cucumbers can be found in packages of six in the produce section of the supermarket.

1 Whisk ¼ cup peanut sauce, lime juice, vinegar and 1 teaspoon oil in large bowl until smooth and well blended. Set aside.

2 Heat remaining 2 teaspoons oil in large nonstick skillet over medium-high heat. Add chicken; cook and stir 4 minutes or until chicken is no longer pink. Remove from heat. Add remaining 2 tablespoons peanut sauce; gently toss to coat evenly.

3 Add lettuce, bell pepper, carrots and cucumber to dressing in large bowl; toss to coat.

4 Divide salad evenly among four plates. Top with chicken, cilantro and peanuts.

Nutrition Information (per serving)

Calories 265, **Total Fat** 10g, **Saturated Fat** 1g, **Cholesterol** 59mg, **Sodium** 643mg, **Carbohydrates** 14g, **Dietary Fiber** 3g, **Protein** 28g

Dietary Exchanges: ½ Bread/Starch • 3 Meat • 1 Vegetable • 1 Fat

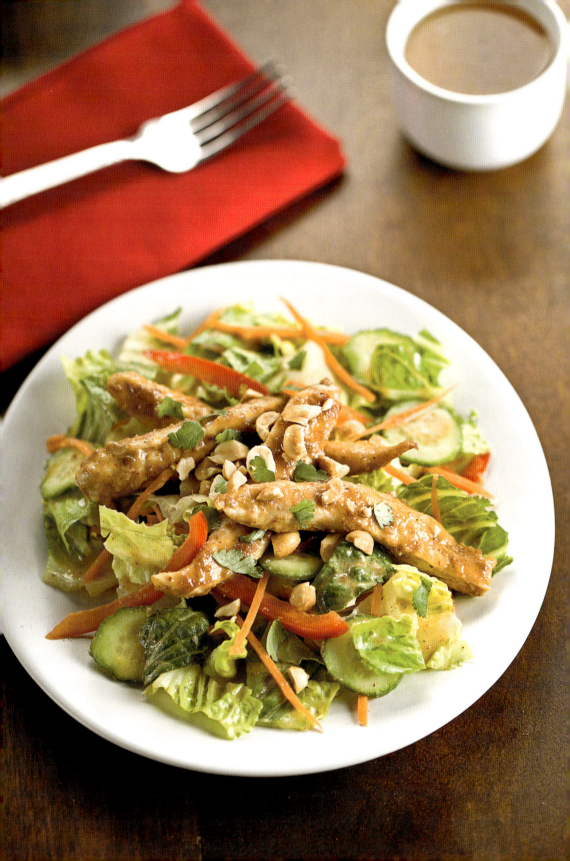

GRILLED STONE FRUIT SALAD

Makes 4 servings

2　tablespoons fresh orange juice

1　tablespoon fresh lemon juice

2　teaspoons canola oil

1　teaspoon honey

½　teaspoon Dijon mustard

1　tablespoon finely chopped fresh mint

1　medium peach, halved and pit removed

1　medium nectarine, halved and pit removed

1　medium plum, halved and pit removed

4　cups mixed baby greens

½　cup crumbled goat cheese

1 Prepare grill for direct cooking over medium-high heat. Spray grid with nonstick cooking spray.

2 Whisk orange juice, lemon juice, oil, honey and mustard in small bowl until smooth and well blended. Stir in mint.

3 Brush cut sides of fruits with orange juice mixture. Set remaining dressing aside. Place fruits, cut sides down, on prepared grid. Grill, covered, 2 to 3 minutes. Turn over; grill 2 to 3 minutes or until fruits begin to soften. Remove to plate; let stand to cool slightly. When cool enough to handle, cut into wedges.

4 Arrange mixed greens on four serving plates. Top evenly with fruits and goat cheese. Drizzle with remaining dressing. Serve immediately.

Nutrition Information (per serving)

Calories 119, **Total Fat** 6g, **Saturated Fat** 3g, **Cholesterol** 11mg, **Sodium** 91mg, **Carbohydrates** 14g, **Dietary Fiber** 2g, **Protein** 4g

Dietary Exchanges: ½ Meat • 1 Fruit • ½ Fat

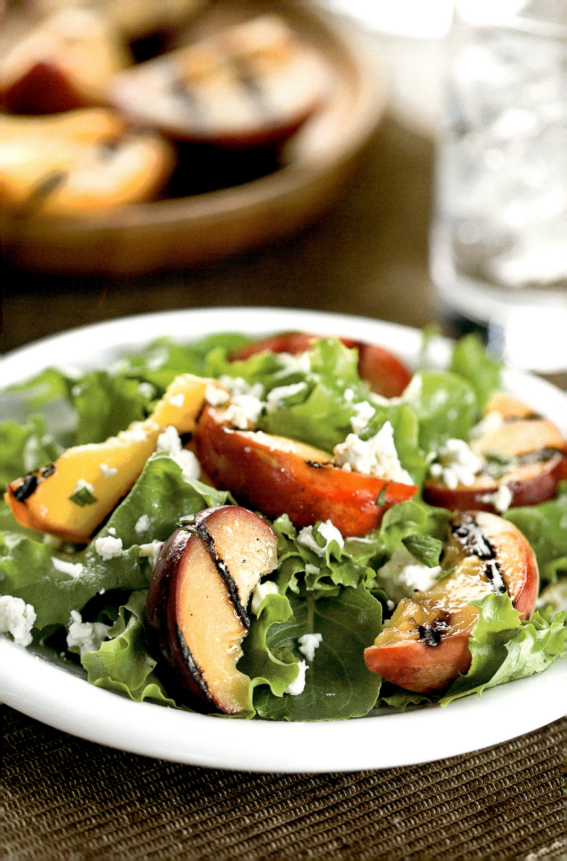

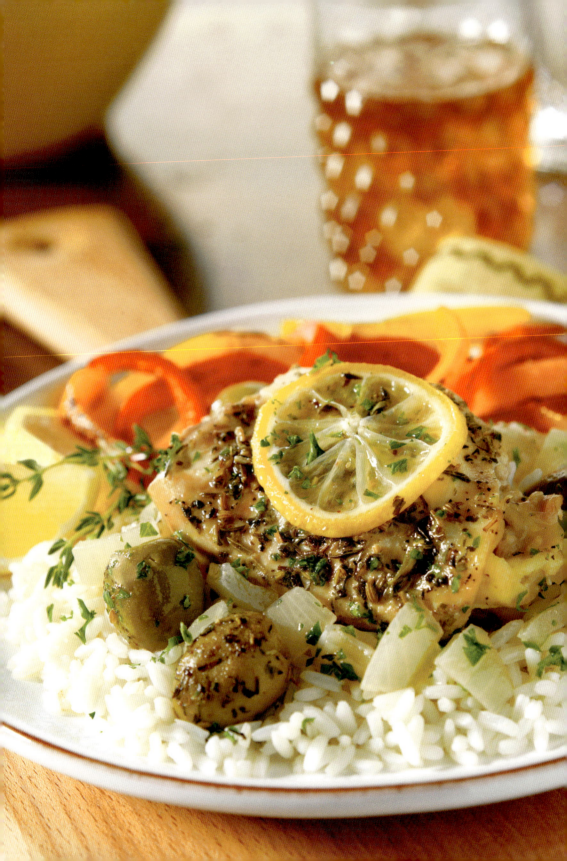

DINNER ENTRÉES

PROVENÇAL LEMON AND OLIVE CHICKEN

Makes 8 servings

- 2 cups chopped onions
- 2 pounds skinless chicken thighs
- 1 medium lemon, thinly sliced and seeded
- ½ cup pitted green olives
- 1 tablespoon white vinegar *or* olive brine
- 2 teaspoons herbes de Provence
- 1 bay leaf
- ½ teaspoon salt
- ⅛ teaspoon black pepper
- 1 cup fat-free reduced-sodium chicken broth
- ½ cup minced fresh parsley

  Hot cooked rice (optional)

SLOW COOKER DIRECTIONS

1 Place onions in slow cooker. Arrange chicken thighs and lemon slices over onions. Add olives, vinegar, herbes de Provence, bay leaf, salt and pepper. Pour in broth.

2 Cover; cook on LOW 5 to 6 hours or on HIGH 3 to 3½ hours or until chicken is tender. Remove and discard bay leaf. Stir in parsley before serving.

3 Serve over rice, if desired.

Nutrition Information (per serving)

Calories 180, **Total Fat** 7g, **Saturated Fat** 1.5g, **Cholesterol** 105mg, **Sodium** 380mg, **Carbohydrates** 5g, **Dietary Fiber** 1g, **Protein** 23g

Dietary Exchanges: 3 Meat • 1 Vegetable • ½ Fat

SKILLET LASAGNA WITH VEGETABLES

Makes 6 servings (1½ cups per serving)

½   **pound hot Italian turkey sausage, casings removed**

½   **pound 93% lean ground turkey**

2   **stalks celery, sliced**

⅓   **cup chopped onion**

2   **cups marinara sauce**

1⅓   **cups water**

4   **ounces uncooked bowtie (farfalle) pasta**

1   **medium zucchini, halved lengthwise and cut into ½-inch-thick slices (2 cups)**

¾   **cup chopped green or yellow bell pepper**

½   **cup reduced-fat ricotta cheese**

2   **tablespoons finely grated Parmesan cheese**

½   **cup (2 ounces) shredded part-skim mozzarella cheese**

1 Cook and stir sausage, turkey, celery and onion in large skillet over medium-high heat until turkey is no longer pink. Stir in marinara sauce and water. Bring to a boil. Add pasta; stir. Reduce heat to medium-low; cover and simmer 12 minutes.

2 Stir in zucchini and bell pepper; cover and simmer 2 minutes. Uncover and simmer 4 to 6 minutes or until vegetables are crisp-tender.

3 Meanwhile, combine ricotta and Parmesan in small bowl. Drop by rounded teaspoonfuls on top of mixture in skillet. Sprinkle with mozzarella. Remove from heat; cover and let stand 10 minutes.

Nutrition Information (per serving)

Calories 300, **Total Fat** 11g, **Saturated Fat** 2.5g, **Cholesterol** 45mg, **Sodium** 750mg, **Carbohydrates** 24g, **Dietary Fiber** 3g, **Protein** 25g

Dietary Exchanges: 1 Bread/Starch • 2½ Meat • ½ Fat

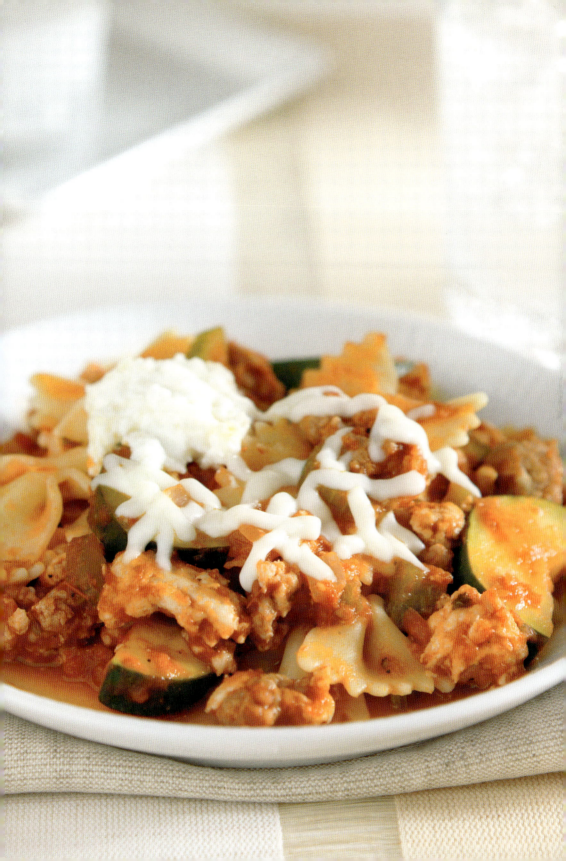

LEMON-GARLIC SALMON WITH TZAZIKI SAUCE

Makes 4 servings

½   **cup diced cucumber**

¾   **teaspoon salt, divided**

1   **cup plain nonfat Greek yogurt**

2   **tablespoons fresh lemon juice, divided**

1   **teaspoon grated lemon peel, divided**

1   **teaspoon minced garlic, divided**

¼   **teaspoon black pepper**

4   **(4-ounce) skinless salmon fillets**

1 Place cucumber in small colander set over small bowl; sprinkle with ¼ teaspoon salt. Drain 1 hour.

2 For Tzaziki Sauce, stir yogurt, cucumber, 1 tablespoon lemon juice, ½ teaspoon lemon peel, ½ teaspoon garlic and ¼ teaspoon salt in small bowl until combined. Cover and refrigerate until ready to use.

3 Combine remaining 1 tablespoon lemon juice, ½ teaspoon lemon peel, ½ teaspoon garlic, ¼ teaspoon salt and pepper in small bowl; mix well. Rub evenly onto salmon.

4 Heat nonstick grill pan over medium-high heat. Cook salmon 5 minutes per side or until fish begins to flake when tested with fork. Serve with Tzaziki Sauce.

SERVING SUGGESTION: Serve this Mediterranean-inspired dish with fresh vegetables or a savory salad, if desired.

Nutrition Information (per serving)

Calories 243, **Total Fat** 12g, **Saturated Fat** 2g, **Cholesterol** 60mg, **Sodium** 508mg, **Carbohydrates** 3g, **Dietary Fiber** 0g, **Protein** 29g

Dietary Exchanges: 3 Meat • 1 Vegetable

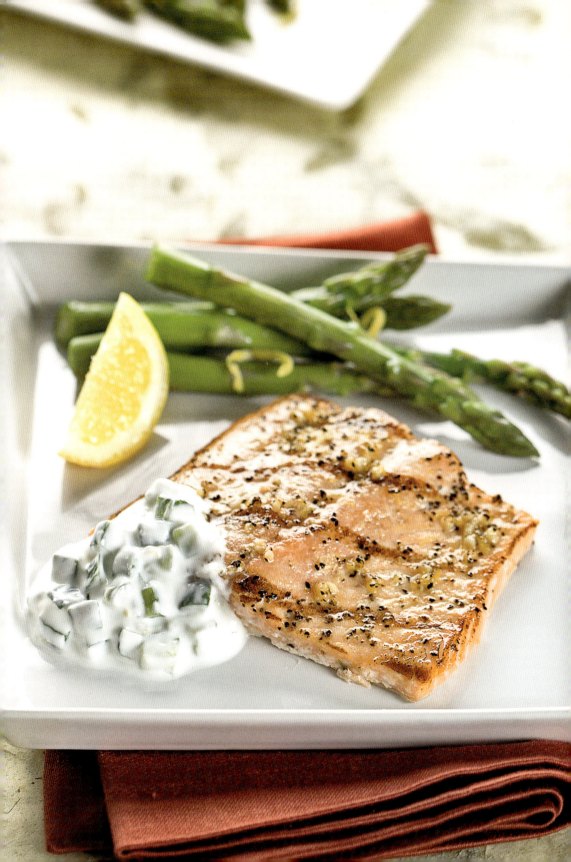

CHICKEN AND VEGGIE FAJITAS

Makes 6 servings

1 pound boneless skinless chicken thighs, cut crosswise into strips

1 teaspoon dried oregano

1 teaspoon chili powder

½ teaspoon garlic salt

2 bell peppers (preferably 1 red and 1 green), cut into thin strips

4 thin slices large sweet or yellow onion, separated into rings

½ cup salsa

6 (6-inch) high-fiber, low-carb flour tortillas, warmed

½ cup chopped fresh cilantro or green onions

Reduced-fat sour cream (optional)

1 Toss chicken with oregano, chili powder and garlic salt in large bowl. Heat large skillet coated with nonstick cooking spray over medium-high heat. Add chicken; cook and stir 5 to 6 minutes or until cooked through. Remove to bowl; set aside.

2 Add bell peppers and onion to same skillet; cook and stir 2 minutes over medium heat. Add salsa; cover and cook 6 to 8 minutes or until vegetables are tender. Uncover; stir in chicken and any juices from bowl. Cook and stir about 2 minutes or until heated through.

3 Serve mixture on top of tortillas topped with cilantro and sour cream, if desired.

Nutrition Information (per serving)

Calories 159, **Total Fat** 5g, **Saturated Fat** 1g, **Cholesterol** 63mg, **Sodium** 476mg, **Carbohydrates** 15g, **Dietary Fiber** 8g, **Protein** 21g

Dietary Exchanges: 1 Bread/Starch • 2 Meat

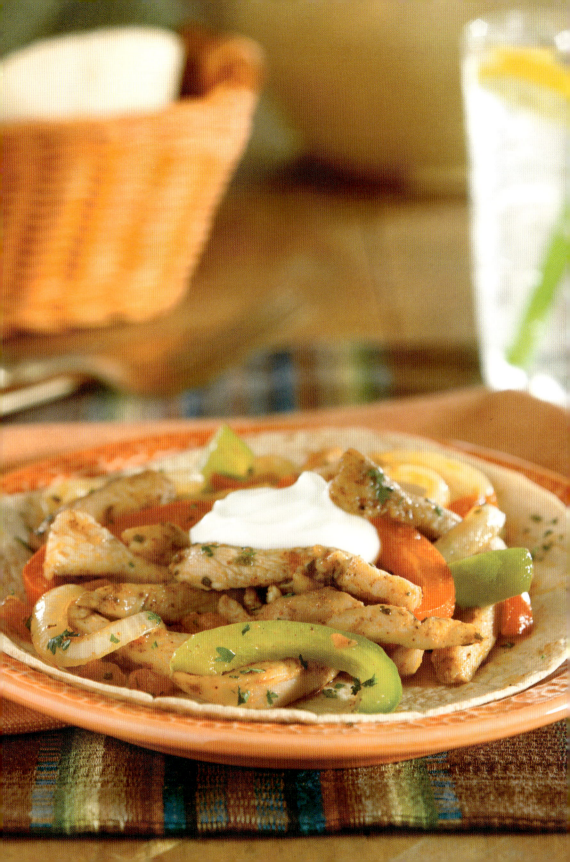

PORK AND TOASTED PEANUT TOSS

Makes 4 servings (1 cup pork mixture and ½ cup rice per serving)

1 packet boil-in-bag rice *or* 1 cup uncooked instant rice

¼ cup plus 2 tablespoons unsalted dry-roasted peanuts

½ pound pork tenderloin, cut into thin strips

3 tablespoons cider vinegar

3 tablespoons reduced-sodium soy sauce

2 tablespoons water

4 packets sugar substitute*

2 teaspoons grated fresh ginger

⅛ teaspoon salt

⅛ teaspoon red pepper flakes

1 medium onion, cut into 8 wedges

1 large green bell pepper, thinly sliced

1 medium carrot, cut into thin strips

This recipe was tested with sucralose-based sugar substitute.

1 Cook rice according to package directions, omitting salt and fat. Set aside.

2 Cook peanuts in large skillet over medium-high heat, stirring constantly, 3 minutes or until lightly browned. Remove to plate; set aside.

3 Spray skillet with nonstick cooking spray. Add pork; cook and stir 3 minutes or until no longer pink. Remove to plate; set aside.

4 Combine vinegar, soy sauce, water, sugar substitute, ginger, salt and red pepper flakes in small saucepan; stir until well blended. Heat over medium heat until warm.

5 Spray skillet with cooking spray. Add onion, bell pepper and carrot; cook and stir 4 minutes or until crisp-tender. Add pork and peanuts to skillet; cook and stir 1 minute.

6 Serve pork mixture over rice; top with sauce.

Nutrition Information (per serving)

Calories 285, **Total Fat** 9g, **Saturated Fat** 2g, **Cholesterol** 37mg, **Sodium** 495mg, **Carbohydrates** 34g, **Dietary Fiber** 3g, **Protein** 19g

Dietary Exchanges: 2 Bread/Starch • 2 Meat • ½ Fat

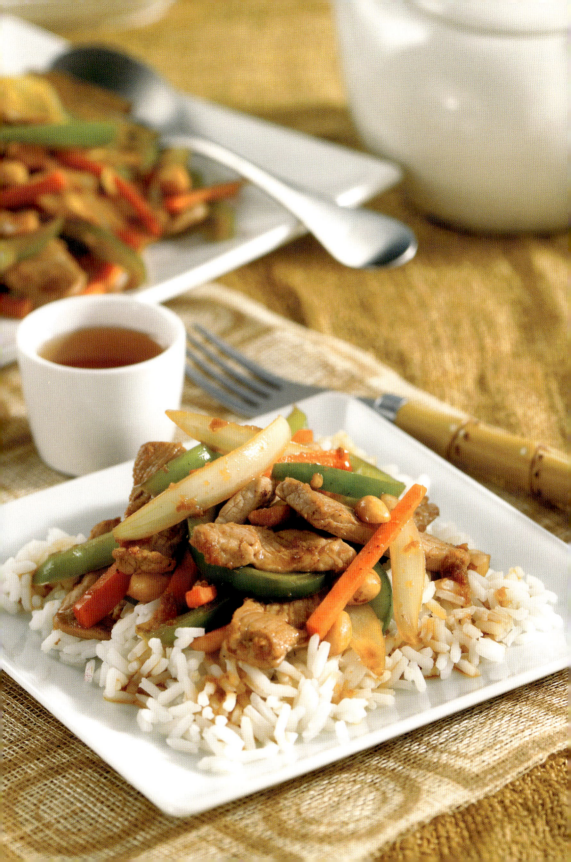

SHRIMP CAPRESE PASTA

Makes 4 servings

1 cup uncooked whole wheat penne

2 teaspoons olive oil

2 cups coarsely chopped grape tomatoes

4 tablespoons chopped fresh basil, divided

1 tablespoon balsamic vinegar

2 cloves garlic, minced

¼ teaspoon salt

⅛ teaspoon red pepper flakes

8 ounces medium raw shrimp, peeled and deveined (with tails on)

1 cup grape tomatoes, halved

2 ounces fresh mozzarella pearls

1 Cook pasta according to package directions, omitting salt. Drain, reserving ½ cup cooking water. Set aside.

2 Heat oil in large skillet over medium heat. Add 2 cups chopped tomatoes, reserved ½ cup pasta water, 2 tablespoons basil, vinegar, garlic, salt and red pepper flakes. Cook and stir 10 minutes or until tomatoes begin to soften.

3 Add shrimp and 1 cup halved tomatoes to skillet; cook and stir 5 minutes or until shrimp turn pink and opaque. Add pasta; cook until heated through.

4 Divide mixture evenly among four bowls. Top evenly with cheese and remaining 2 tablespoons basil.

Nutrition Information (per serving)

Calories 222, **Total Fat** 6g, **Saturated Fat** 2g, **Cholesterol** 81mg, **Sodium** 550mg, **Carbohydrates** 27g, **Dietary Fiber** 4g, **Protein** 17g

Dietary Exchanges: 1½ Bread/Starch • 1½ Meat • 1 Vegetable

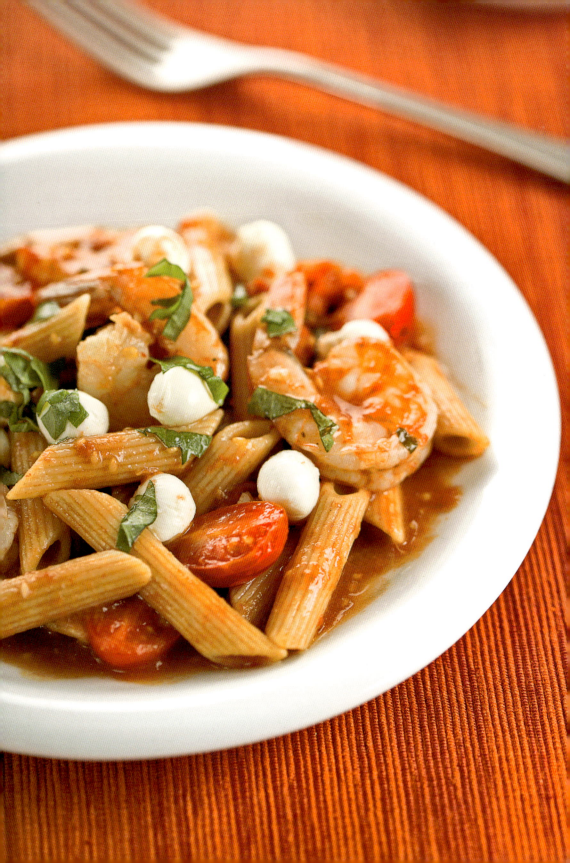

EASY MAKE-AT-HOME CHINESE CHICKEN

Makes 4 servings

3 tablespoons frozen orange juice concentrate, thawed

2 tablespoons water

2 tablespoons reduced-sodium soy sauce

¾ teaspoon cornstarch

¼ teaspoon garlic powder

2 carrots, sliced

1 package (12 ounces) frozen broccoli and cauliflower florets, thawed

2 teaspoons canola oil

¾ pound boneless skinless chicken breasts, cut into bite-size pieces

1⅓ cups hot cooked rice

1 For sauce, stir together orange juice concentrate, water, soy sauce, cornstarch and garlic powder; set aside.

2 Spray nonstick wok or large skillet with nonstick cooking spray. Add carrots; stir-fry over high heat 1 minute. Add broccoli and cauliflower; stir-fry 2 to 3 minutes or until vegetables are crisp-tender. Remove vegetables from wok; set aside.

3 Add oil to wok; heat over medium-high heat. Stir-fry chicken in hot oil 2 to 3 minutes or until cooked through. Push chicken up side of wok. Stir sauce; add to wok. Bring to a boil. Return vegetables to wok; cook and stir until heated through. Serve over rice.

TIP: To cut carrots decoratively, use a citrus stripper or grapefruit spoon to cut 4 or 5 grooves into whole carrots, cutting lengthwise from stem end to tip. Then cut carrots crosswise into slices.

Nutrition Information (per serving)

Calories 215, **Total Fat** 3g, **Saturated Fat** 1g, **Cholesterol** 32mg, **Sodium** 351mg, **Carbohydrates** 29g, **Dietary Fiber** 4g, **Protein** 18g

Dietary Exchanges: 1 Bread/Starch • 2 Meat • 2 Vegetable

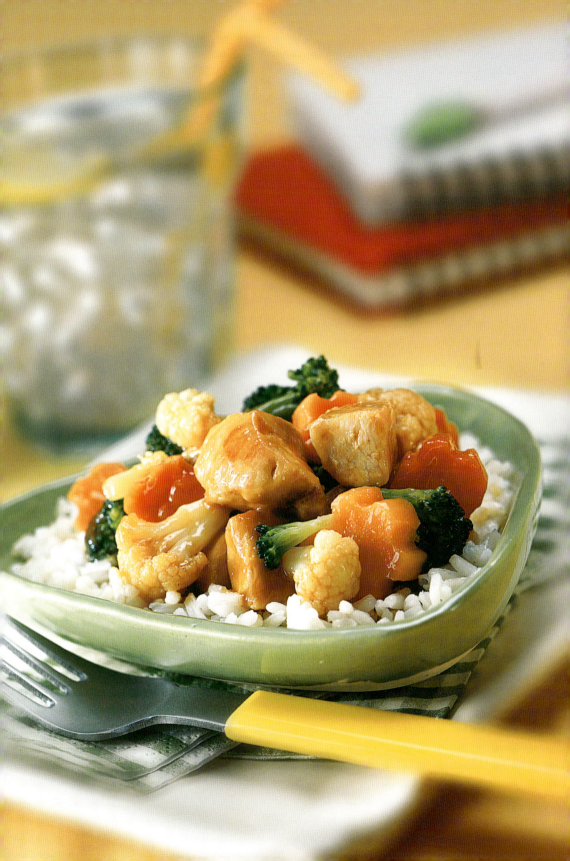

BALSAMIC CHICKEN

Makes 6 servings

1½   teaspoons fresh rosemary leaves, minced, *or* ½ teaspoon dried rosemary

2   cloves garlic, minced

¾   teaspoon black pepper

½   teaspoon salt

6   boneless skinless chicken breasts (about ¼ pound each)

1   tablespoon olive oil

¼   cup balsamic vinegar

1 Combine rosemary, garlic, pepper and salt in small bowl; mix well. Place chicken in large bowl; drizzle chicken with oil and rub with spice mixture. Cover and refrigerate several hours.

2 Preheat oven to 450°F. Spray heavy roasting pan or cast iron skillet with nonstick cooking spray. Place chicken in pan; bake 10 minutes. Turn chicken over, stirring in 3 to 4 tablespoons water if drippings begin to stick to pan.

3 Bake about 10 minutes or until chicken is golden brown and no longer pink in center. If pan is dry, stir in another 1 to 2 tablespoons water to loosen drippings.

4 Drizzle vinegar over chicken in pan. Remove chicken to plates. Stir liquid in pan; drizzle over chicken.

Nutrition Information (per serving)

Calories 174, **Total Fat** 5g, **Saturated Fat** 1g, **Cholesterol** 73mg, **Sodium** 242mg, **Carbohydrates** 3g, **Dietary Fiber** 1g, **Protein** 27g

Dietary Exchanges: 3 Meat

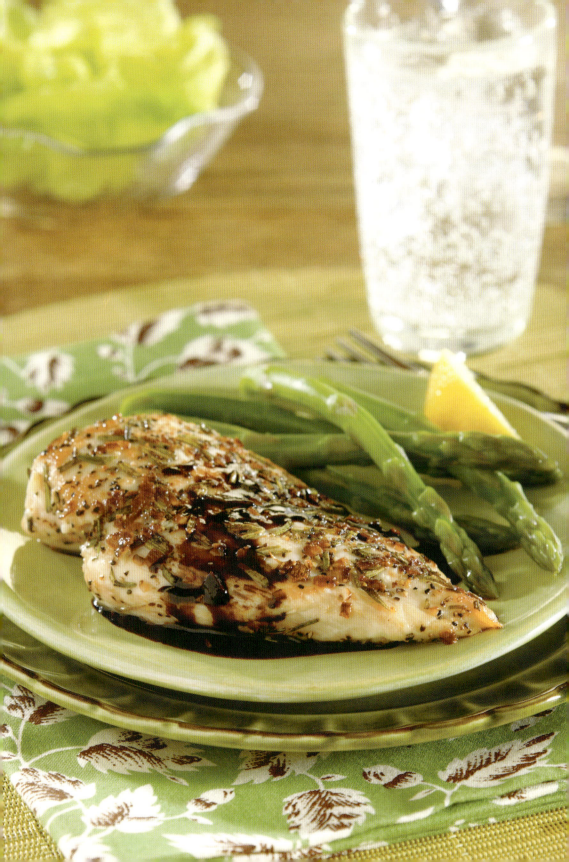

GRILLED HALIBUT WITH CHERRY TOMATO RELISH

Makes 4 servings (1 fish fillet and ½ cup relish per serving)

3   tablespoons fresh lemon juice, divided

2   teaspoons grated lemon peel, divided

2   cloves garlic, minced

2   teaspoons olive oil, divided

¼   teaspoon salt, divided

¼   teaspoon black pepper, divided

4   halibut fillets (about 6 ounces each)

2   cups cherry tomatoes, quartered

2   tablespoons chopped fresh parsley

1 Combine 2 tablespoons lemon juice, 1 teaspoon lemon peel, garlic, 1 teaspoon oil, ⅛ teaspoon salt and ⅛ teaspoon pepper in large resealable food storage bag. Add halibut; seal bag and refrigerate 1 hour.

2 Combine tomatoes, parsley, remaining 1 tablespoon lemon juice, 1 teaspoon lemon peel, 1 teaspoon oil, ⅛ teaspoon salt and ⅛ teaspoon pepper in medium bowl; set aside.

3 Prepare grill for direct cooking. Spray grid with nonstick cooking spray.

4 Remove halibut from marinade; discard marinade. Place halibut on prepared grid; grill 3 to 5 minutes per side or until fish begins to flake when tested with fork. Serve with relish.

Nutrition Information (per serving)

Calories 215, **Total Fat** 5g, **Saturated Fat** 1g, **Cholesterol** 54mg, **Sodium** 185mg, **Carbohydrates** 4g, **Dietary Fiber** 1g, **Protein** 28g

Dietary Exchanges: 4 Meat • 1 Vegetable

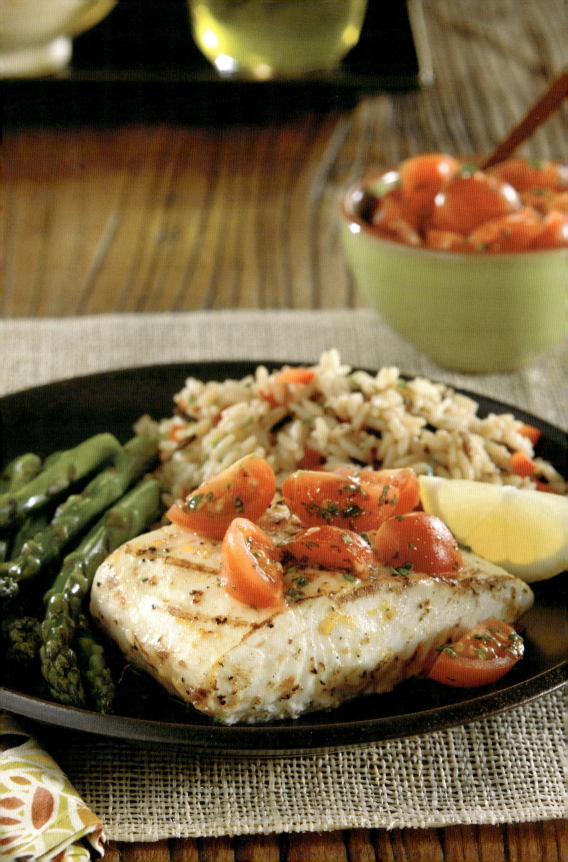

ROASTED SALMON WITH STRAWBERRY-ORANGE SALSA

Makes 4 servings (1 salmon fillet and ⅓ cup salsa per serving)

4   salmon fillets (about ¼ pound each), skin removed

½   teaspoon ground cumin

½   teaspoon dried thyme

¼   teaspoon salt

¼   teaspoon black pepper

1   medium orange

1   cup diced fresh strawberries

¼   cup finely chopped poblano pepper* or green bell pepper

2   tablespoons finely chopped fresh cilantro

½   teaspoon grated fresh ginger

Poblano peppers can sting and irritate the skin, so wear rubber gloves when handling peppers and do not touch your eyes.

1 Preheat oven to 400°F.

2 Line baking sheet with foil; spray with nonstick cooking spray. Place salmon on prepared baking sheet; sprinkle with cumin, thyme, salt and black pepper. Bake 12 to 14 minutes or until salmon begins to flake when tested with fork.

3 Meanwhile, grate orange peel to measure ½ teaspoon; place in medium bowl. Peel and section orange; coarsely chop orange sections. Add orange sections, strawberries, poblano pepper, cilantro and ginger to bowl; mix well. Serve salmon with salsa.

Nutrition Information (per serving)

Calories 241, **Total Fat** 12g, **Saturated Fat** 2g, **Cholesterol** 66mg, **Sodium** 214mg, **Carbohydrates** 8g, **Dietary Fiber** 2g, **Protein** 24g

Dietary Exchanges: 3 Meat • ½ Fruit • 1 Fat

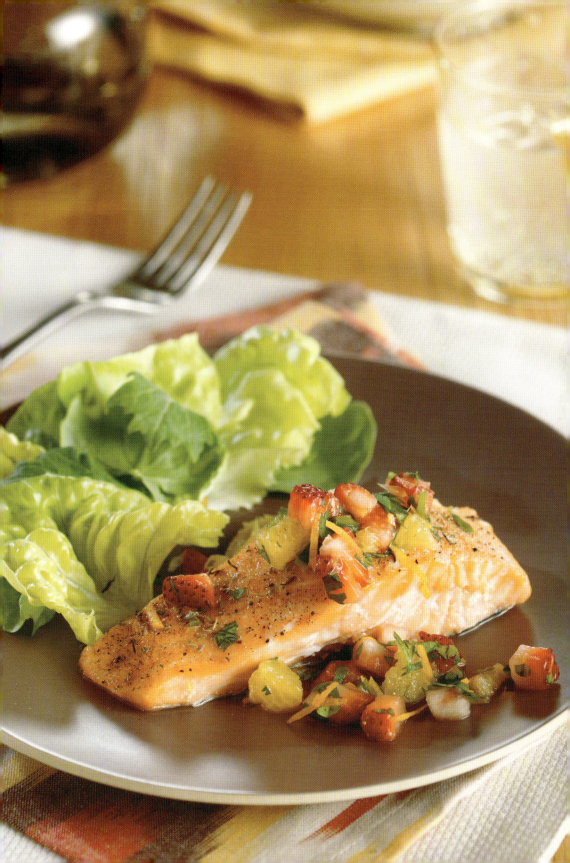

ORANGE CHICKEN STIR-FRY OVER QUINOA

Makes 4 servings (1 cup chicken mixture and ⅓ cup quinoa per serving)

½ cup uncooked quinoa

1 cup water

2 teaspoons vegetable oil, divided

1 pound boneless skinless chicken breasts, cut into thin strips

1 cup fresh squeezed orange juice (2 to 3 oranges)

1 tablespoon reduced-sodium soy sauce

1 tablespoon cornstarch

½ cup sliced green onions

2 tablespoons grated fresh ginger

6 ounces snow peas, ends trimmed

1 cup thinly sliced carrots

¼ teaspoon red pepper flakes (optional)

1 Place quinoa in fine-mesh strainer; rinse well under cold running water. Bring 1 cup water to a boil in medium saucepan; stir in quinoa. Reduce heat to low; cover and simmer 10 to 15 minutes or until quinoa is tender and water is absorbed.

2 Meanwhile, heat 1 teaspoon oil in large skillet over medium-high heat. Add chicken; cook and stir 4 to 6 minutes or until no longer pink. Remove to plate; keep warm.

3 Stir orange juice and soy sauce into cornstarch in small bowl until smooth; set aside. Heat remaining 1 teaspoon oil in skillet. Add green onions and ginger; stir-fry 1 to 2 minutes. Add snow peas and carrots; stir-fry 4 to 5 minutes or until carrots are crisp-tender.

4 Return chicken to skillet. Stir orange juice mixture; add to skillet. Bring to a boil. Reduce heat; simmer until slightly thickened.

5 Serve chicken and vegetables over quinoa; sprinkle with red pepper flakes, if desired.

Nutrition Information (per serving)

Calories 149, **Total Fat** 3g, **Saturated Fat** 1g, **Cholesterol** 33mg, **Sodium** 119mg, **Carbohydrates** 15g, **Dietary Fiber** 2g, **Protein** 16g

Dietary Exchanges: 1 Bread/Starch • 2 Meat

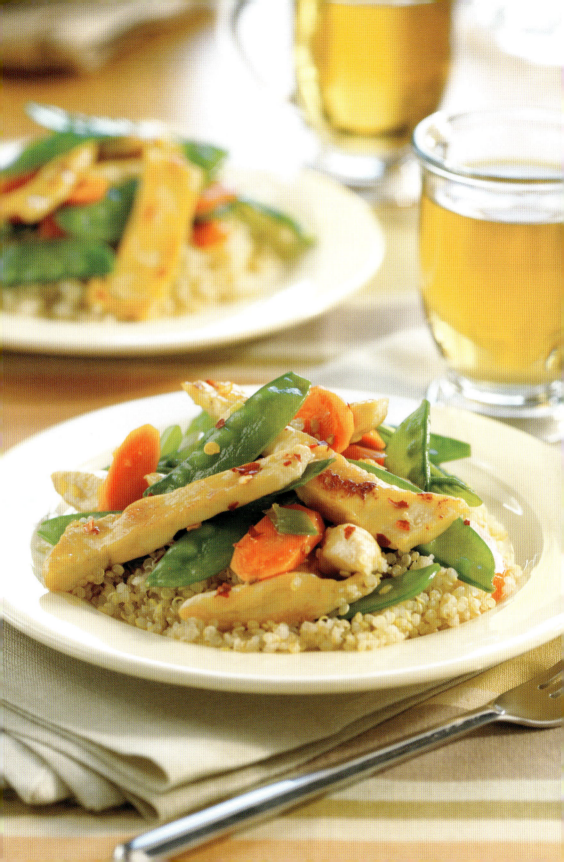

CHICKEN MIRABELLA

Makes 4 servings

4   boneless skinless chicken breasts (about 4 ounces each)

½   cup pitted prunes

½   cup assorted pitted olives (black, green and/or a combination)

¼   cup light white grape juice or dry white wine

2   tablespoons olive oil

1   tablespoon capers

1   tablespoon red wine vinegar

1   teaspoon dried oregano

1   clove garlic, minced

½   teaspoon chopped fresh parsley, plus additional for garnish

2   teaspoons packed brown sugar

1 Preheat oven to 350°F.

2 Place chicken in 8-inch baking dish. Combine prunes, olives, grape juice, oil, capers, vinegar, oregano, garlic and ½ teaspoon parsley in medium bowl. Pour evenly over chicken. Sprinkle with brown sugar.

3 Bake 25 to 30 minutes or until chicken is no longer pink in center, basting with sauce halfway through. Garnish with additional parsley.

TIP: For more intense flavor, marinate chicken at least 8 hours or overnight and sprinkle with brown sugar just before baking.

SERVING SUGGESTION: Serve with long grain and wild rice which offers protein, fiber, and many minerals, including iron, and some vitamins.

Nutrition Information (per serving)

Calories 280, **Total Fat** 11g, **Saturated Fat** 2g, **Cholesterol** 72mg, **Sodium** 291mg, **Carbohydrates** 20g, **Dietary Fiber** 2g, **Protein** 25g

Dietary Exchanges: 3 Meat • 1 Fruit • 1 Fat

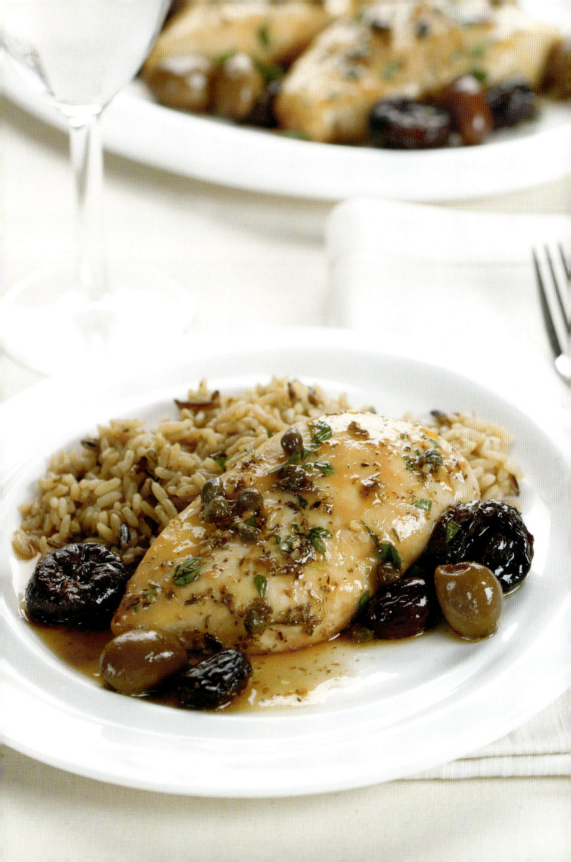

HOLIDAY STUFFED BEEF TENDERLOIN

Makes 8 servings

- 4 teaspoons olive oil, divided
- 2 shallots, minced
- 1 package (8 ounces) sliced cremini mushrooms
- 3 cloves garlic, minced and divided
- 1 tablespoon chopped fresh thyme, plus additional for garnish
- 1½ teaspoons chopped fresh parsley, plus additional for garnish
- ¼ cup dry sherry or red wine vinegar
- 2 to 3 pounds beef tenderloin
- ½ cup fresh whole wheat bread crumbs*
- 1 teaspoon salt
- ½ teaspoon black pepper

To make fresh bread crumbs, tear 1 slice bread into pieces; process in food processor until coarse crumbs form.

1 Preheat oven to 425°F.

2 Heat 2 teaspoons oil in large skillet over medium heat. Add shallots; cook and stir 5 minutes or until tender. Add mushrooms, cook and stir 8 minutes or until softened. Stir in 1 clove garlic, 1 tablespoon thyme and 1½ teaspoons parsley; cook and stir 1 minute.

3 Pour sherry into skillet. Bring to a boil over medium heat; boil 2 minutes or until sherry is reduced by about half. Cool slightly.

4 Cut beef tenderloin lengthwise. (Do not cut all the way through). Open up beef; cover with plastic or waxed paper. Pound using meat mallet to ½-inch thickness.

5 Stir bread crumbs into mushroom mixture; spread evenly onto center of beef, leaving 1-inch border around edges. Roll up beef jelly-roll style. Secure with kitchen string at 1-inch intervals. Place beef on rack in shallow roasting pan.

6 Combine remaining 2 teaspoons oil, 2 cloves garlic, salt and pepper in small bowl. Rub mixture evenly over beef.

7 Roast 35 to 40 minutes for medium rare (135°F) or until desired doneness is reached. Remove roast to carving board; tent loosely with foil. Let stand 15 to 20 minutes before carving and serving. Sprinkle with additional thyme and parsley, if desired.

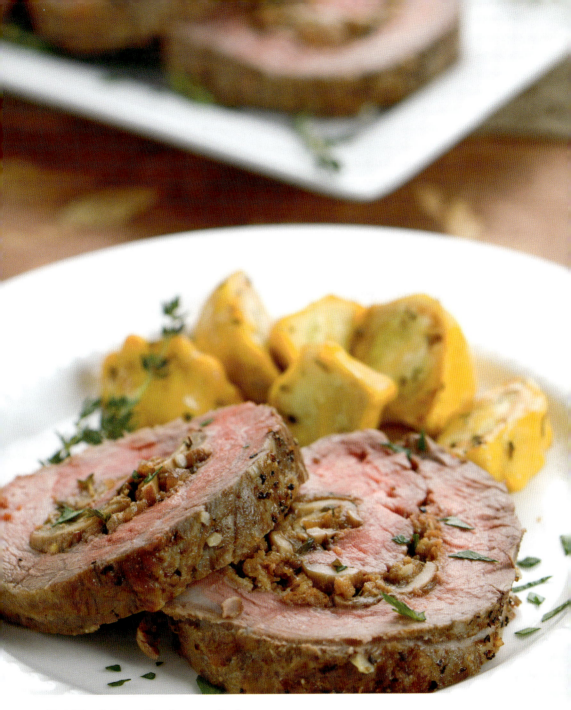

Nutrition Information (per serving)

Calories 195, **Total Fat** 9g, **Saturated Fat** 3g, **Cholesterol** 59mg, **Sodium** 381mg, **Carbohydrates** 5g, **Dietary Fiber** 1g, **Protein** 21g

Dietary Exchanges: ½ Bread/Starch • 3 Meat

RED SNAPPER VERA CRUZ

Makes 4 servings (1 fish fillet and ½ cup salsa per serving)

4   red snapper fillets (about 1 pound)

¼   cup fresh lime juice

1   tablespoon fresh lemon juice

1   teaspoon chili powder

4   green onions with 4 inches of tops, sliced into ½-inch lengths

1   tomato, coarsely chopped

½   cup chopped Anaheim or green bell pepper

½   cup chopped red bell pepper

Black pepper

MICROWAVE DIRECTIONS

1 Place red snapper in shallow 9- to 10-inch round microwavable baking dish. Combine lime juice, lemon juice and chili powder in small bowl. Pour over snapper. Marinate 10 minutes, turning once or twice.

2 Sprinkle green onions, tomato, Anaheim and bell pepper over snapper. Season with black pepper. Cover dish loosely with vented plastic wrap. Microwave on HIGH 5 to 6 minutes or just until snapper flakes in center, rotating dish every 2 minutes. Let stand, covered, 4 minutes.

NOTE: Serve over hot cooked rice, if desired.

Nutrition Information (per serving)

Calories 144, **Total Fat** 2g, **Saturated Fat** 1g, **Cholesterol** 42mg, **Sodium** 61mg, **Carbohydrates** 7g, **Dietary Fiber** 2g, **Protein** 24g

Dietary Exchanges: 2½ Meat • 1 Vegetable

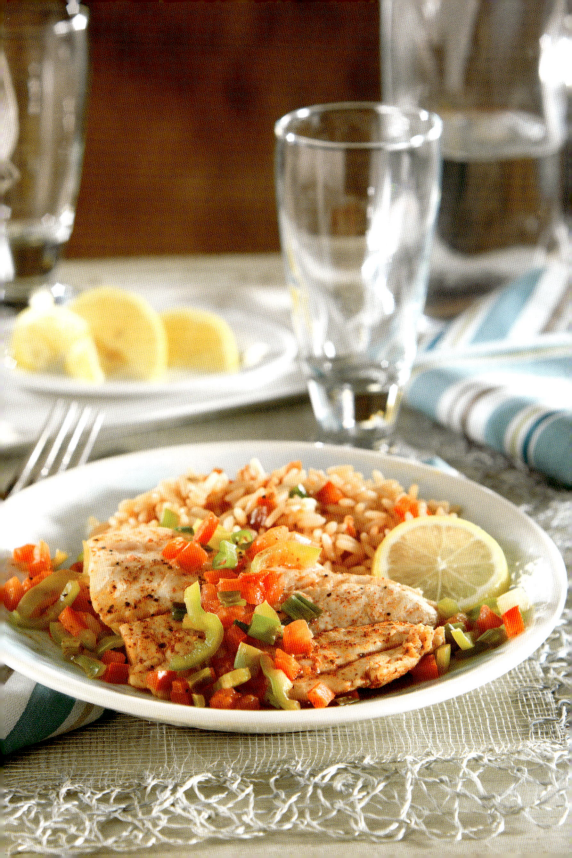

MEDITERRANEAN CHICKEN KABOBS

Makes 8 servings (2 kabobs per serving)

2 pounds boneless skinless chicken breasts or chicken tenders, cut into 1-inch pieces

1 small eggplant, peeled and cut into 1-inch pieces

1 medium zucchini, cut crosswise into ½-inch slices

2 medium onions, each cut into 8 wedges

16 medium mushrooms, stemmed

16 cherry tomatoes

1 cup fat-free, reduced-sodium chicken broth

⅔ cup balsamic vinegar

3 tablespoons olive oil

2 tablespoons dried mint

4 teaspoons dried basil

1 tablespoon dried oregano

1 Alternately thread chicken, eggplant, zucchini, onions, mushrooms and tomatoes onto 16 metal skewers; place in large glass baking dish.

2 Combine broth, vinegar, oil, mint, basil and oregano in small bowl; pour over kabobs. Cover and marinate in refrigerator 2 hours, turning kabobs occasionally. Remove kabobs from marinade; discard marinade.

3 Preheat broiler. Broil kabobs 6 inches from heat 10 to 15 minutes or until chicken is cooked through, turning kabobs halfway through cooking time.

NOTE: Serve over couscous, if desired.

Nutrition Information (per serving)

Calories 200, **Total Fat** 7g, **Saturated Fat** 1g, **Cholesterol** 50mg, **Sodium** 300mg, **Carbohydrates** 11g, **Dietary Fiber** 3g, **Protein** 25g

Dietary Exchanges: 3 Meat • 2 Vegetable • 1 Fat

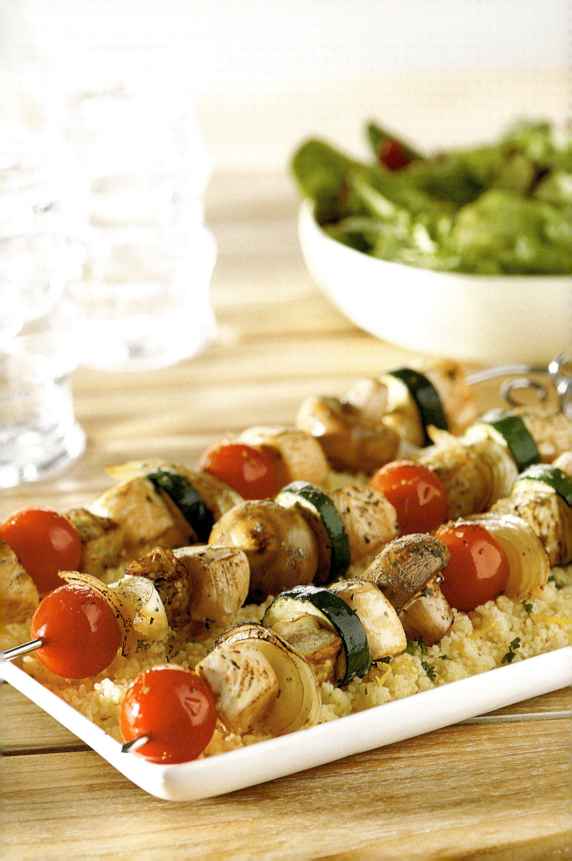

GREEK CHICKEN BURGERS WITH CUCUMBER YOGURT SAUCE

Makes 4 servings (1 [4-ounce] burger and ¼ of sauce per serving)

½ cup plus 2 tablespoons plain nonfat Greek yogurt

½ medium cucumber, peeled, seeded and finely chopped

Juice of ½ lemon

3 cloves garlic, minced, divided

2 teaspoons finely chopped fresh mint *or* ½ teaspoon dried mint

⅛ teaspoon salt

⅛ teaspoon ground white pepper

1 pound ground chicken breast

3 ounces reduced-fat crumbled feta cheese

4 large kalamata olives, rinsed, patted dry and minced

1 egg

½ to 1 teaspoon dried oregano

¼ teaspoon black pepper

Mixed baby lettuce (optional)

Fresh mint leaves (optional)

1 Combine yogurt, cucumber, lemon juice, 2 cloves garlic, 2 teaspoons mint, salt and white pepper in medium bowl; mix well. Cover and refrigerate until ready to serve.

2 Combine chicken, cheese, olives, egg, oregano, black pepper and remaining 1 clove garlic in large bowl; mix well. Shape mixture into four patties.

3 Spray grill pan with nonstick cooking spray; heat over medium-high heat. Grill patties 5 to 7 minutes per side or until cooked through (165°F).

4 Serve burgers with sauce and mixed greens, if desired. Garnish with mint leaves.

Nutrition Information (per serving)

Calories 260, **Total Fat** 14g, **Saturated Fat** 5g, **Cholesterol** 150mg, **Sodium** 500mg, **Carbohydrates** 4g, **Dietary Fiber** 1g, **Protein** 29g

Dietary Exchanges: 3 Meat • ½ Vegetable • 1 Fat

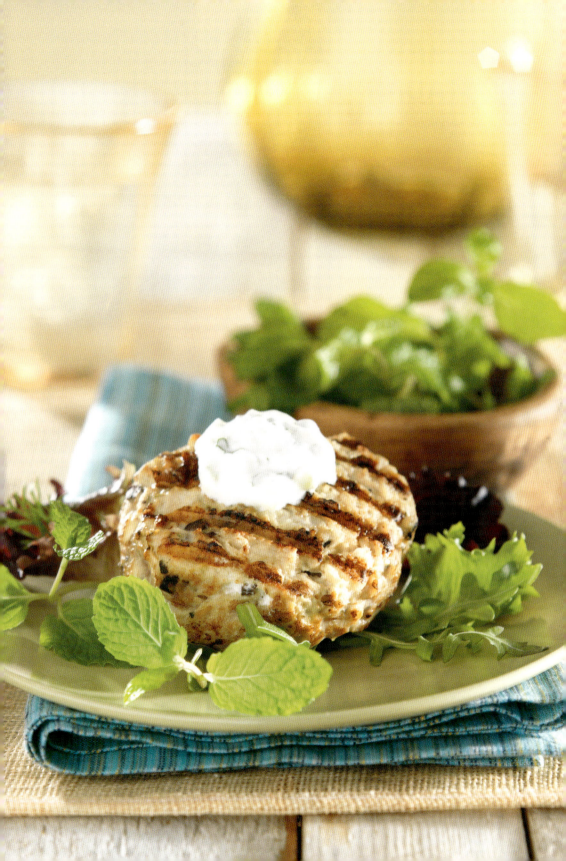

SHRIMP AND AVOCADO TOSTADAS

Makes 4 servings

1 cup canned low-fat refried black beans

8 ounces medium raw shrimp, peeled and deveined

3 cloves garlic, minced

3 green onions, sliced

½ cup salsa

1 ripe avocado, diced

4 tostada shells, warmed

½ cup shredded romaine lettuce

½ cup diced tomato

1 Heat small saucepan over medium heat; add refried beans and cook until heated through.

2 Meanwhile, spray large nonstick skillet with nonstick cooking spray; heat over medium-high heat. Add shrimp and garlic; cook and stir 3 minutes or until shrimp are pink and opaque. Add green onions; cook and stir 30 seconds. Stir in salsa; cook until heated through. Remove from heat; gently stir in avocado.

3 Spread beans evenly over tostada shells; top with shrimp mixture, lettuce and tomato.

Nutrition Information (per serving)

Calories 214, **Total Fat** 10g, **Saturated Fat** 2g, **Cholesterol** 86mg, **Sodium** 430mg, **Carbohydrates** 18g, **Dietary Fiber** 5g, **Protein** 15g

Dietary Exchanges: 1 Bread/Starch • 1 Meat • 1 Vegetable • 1½ Fat

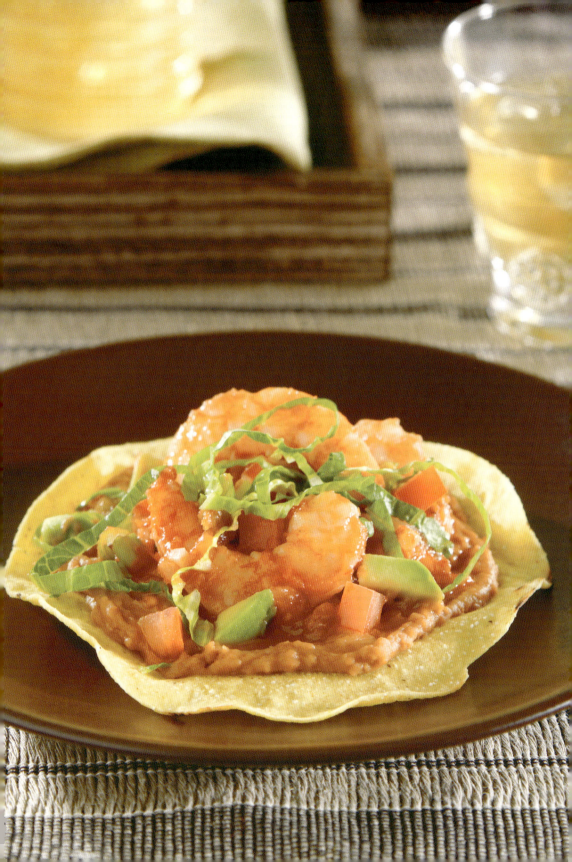

BALSAMIC GRILLED PORK CHOPS

Makes 2 servings (3 ounces pork and 1½ teaspoons sauce per serving)

- 2 tablespoons balsamic vinegar
- 2 tablespoons reduced-sodium soy sauce
- 1 teaspoon Dijon mustard
- 2 teaspoons sugar
- ⅛ teaspoon red pepper flakes
- 2 boneless pork chops, trimmed of fat (8 ounces total)

1 Combine vinegar, soy sauce, mustard, sugar and red pepper flakes in small bowl. Stir until well blended. Reserve 1 tablespoon marinade; refrigerate until needed.

2 Place pork in large resealable food storage bag. Pour remaining marinade over pork. Seal bag; turn to coat. Refrigerate 2 hours or up to 24 hours.

3 Spray grill pan with nonstick cooking spray; heat over medium-high heat. Remove pork from marinade; discard marinade. Cook pork 4 minutes on each side or until just slightly pink in center. Place on plates; top with reserved 1 tablespoon marinade.

Nutrition Information (per serving)

Calories 196, **Total Fat** 5g, **Saturated Fat** 2g, **Cholesterol** 63mg, **Sodium** 653mg, **Carbohydrates** 8g, **Dietary Fiber** 1g, **Protein** 26g

Dietary Exchanges: 1½ Bread/Starch • 3 Meat

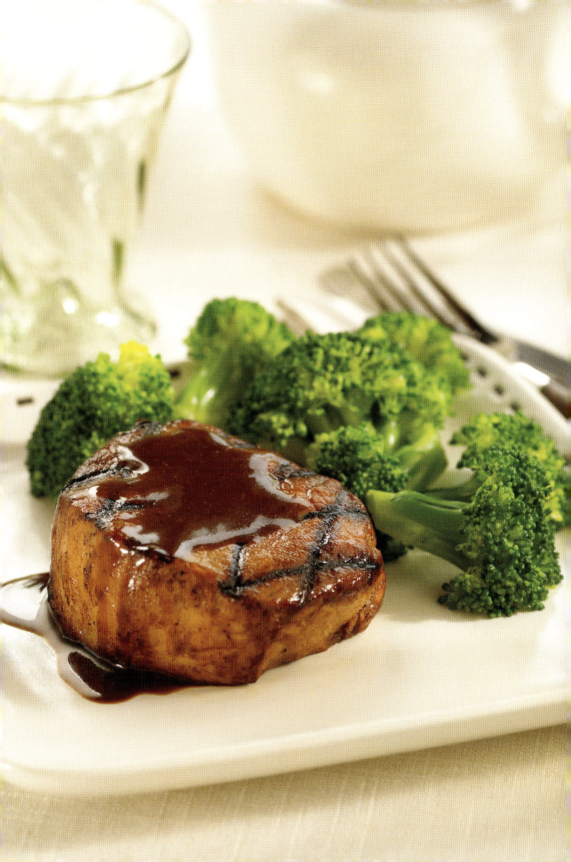

GRILLED SALSA TURKEY BURGER

Makes 1 serving

3 ounces 93% lean ground turkey

1 tablespoon mild or medium salsa

1 tablespoon crushed baked tortilla chips

1 slice (1 ounce) reduced-fat Monterey Jack cheese (optional)

1 whole wheat hamburger bun, split

Green leaf lettuce

Additional salsa (optional)

1 Prepare grill for direct cooking. Lightly spray grid with nonstick cooking spray.

2 Combine turkey, salsa and chips in small bowl; mix lightly. Shape into patty.

3 Grill burger over medium-high heat about 6 minutes per side or until cooked through (165°F). Top with cheese, if desired, during last 2 minutes of grilling. Toast bun on grill, cut sides down, during last 2 minutes of grilling.

4 Place lettuce on bottom half of bun; top with burger, additional salsa, if desired, and top half of bun.

NOTE: To broil, preheat broiler. Broil burger 4 to 6 inches from heat 6 minutes per side or until cooked through (165°F).

Nutrition Information (per serving)

Calories 302, **Total Fat** 11g, **Saturated Fat** 3g, **Cholesterol** 63mg, **Sodium** 494mg, **Carbohydrates** 29g, **Dietary Fiber** 2g, **Protein** 22g

Dietary Exchanges: 2 Bread/Starch • 2 Meat • 1 Fat

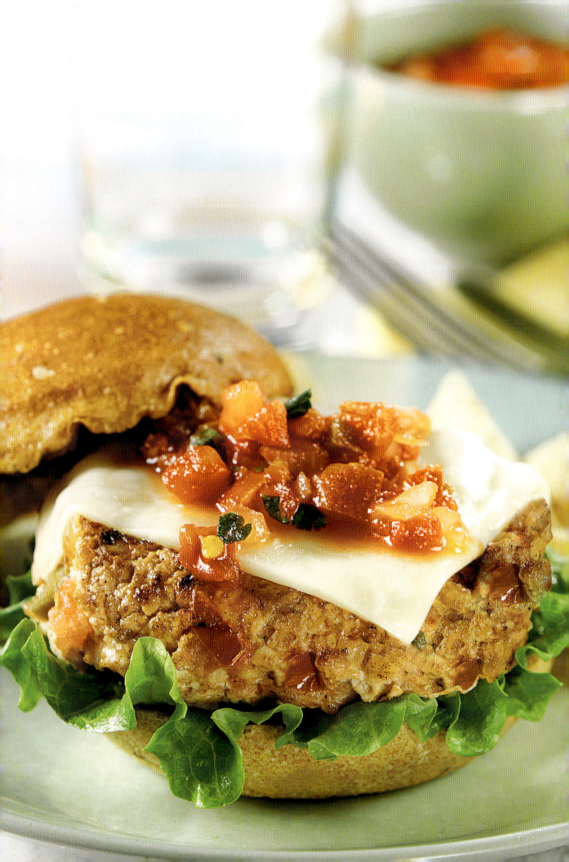

CHICKEN & WILD RICE SKILLET DINNER

Makes 1 serving

1 teaspoon reduced-fat margarine

2 ounces boneless skinless chicken breast, cut into strips (about ½ chicken breast)

1 package (5 ounces) long grain and wild rice mix with seasoning

½ cup water

3 dried apricots, cut up

1 Melt margarine in small skillet over medium-high heat. Add chicken; cook and stir 3 to 5 minutes or until cooked through.

2 Meanwhile, measure ¼ cup of the rice and 1 tablespoon plus ½ teaspoon of the seasoning mix. Reserve remaining rice and seasoning mix for another use.

3 Add rice, seasoning mix, water and apricots to skillet; mix well. Bring to a boil. Cover and reduce heat to low; simmer 25 minutes or until liquid is absorbed and rice is tender.

Nutrition Information (per serving)

Calories 314, **Total Fat** 5g, **Saturated Fat** 1g, **Cholesterol** 52mg, **Sodium** 669mg, **Carbohydrates** 44g, **Dietary Fiber** 3g, **Protein** 24g

Dietary Exchanges: 3 Bread/Starch • 2 Meat

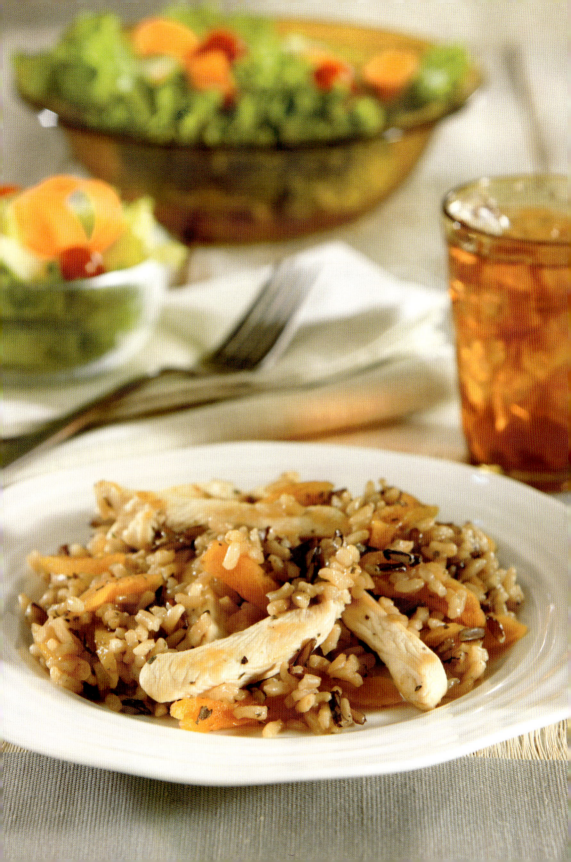

MINI MEATLOAVES

Makes 6 servings (1 meatloaf per serving)

3 tablespoons ketchup

1 tablespoon balsamic vinegar

1 tablespoon olive oil

1½ cups finely chopped onion

1½ cups finely chopped mushrooms

1½ cups chopped baby spinach

1½ pounds extra lean ground sirloin

¾ cup old-fashioned oats

2 egg whites

½ teaspoon salt

½ teaspoon black pepper

1 Preheat oven to 375°F. Spray 6 mini (4¼×2½-inch) loaf pans with nonstick cooking spray. Whisk ketchup and vinegar in small bowl until smooth and well blended; set aside.

2 Heat oil in large skillet over medium heat. Add onion, mushrooms and spinach; cook and stir 8 minutes or until tender. Remove to large bowl. Let stand until cool enough to handle.

3 Add beef, oats, egg whites, salt and pepper to vegetables; mix well. Divide mixture evenly among prepared pans. Brush half of ketchup mixture evenly over loaves.

4 Bake 15 minutes. Brush with remaining ketchup mixture. Bake 5 minutes or until cooked through (160°F).

Nutrition Information (per serving)

Calories 270, **Total Fat** 11g, **Saturated Fat** 3g, **Cholesterol** 62mg, **Sodium** 362mg, **Carbohydrates** 14g, **Dietary Fiber** 2g, **Protein** 28g

Dietary Exchanges: 1 Bread/Starch • 3½ Meat

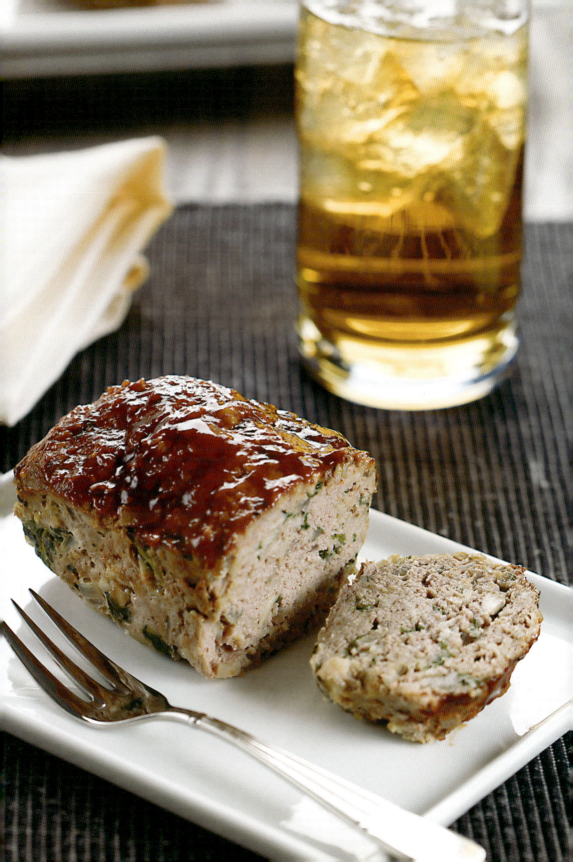

GREEK-STYLE BEEF KABOBS

Makes 4 servings (1 kabob per serving)

1 pound beef top sirloin steak (1 inch thick), cut into 16 pieces

¼ cup fat-free Italian salad dressing

3 tablespoons fresh lemon juice, divided

1 tablespoon dried oregano

1 tablespoon Worcestershire sauce

2 teaspoons dried basil

1 teaspoon grated lemon peel

⅛ teaspoon red pepper flakes

1 large green bell pepper, cut into 16 pieces

16 cherry tomatoes

2 teaspoons olive oil

⅛ teaspoon salt

1 Combine beef, salad dressing, 2 tablespoons lemon juice, oregano, Worcestershire sauce, basil, lemon peel and red pepper flakes in large resealable food storage bag. Seal bag; turn to coat. Marinate in refrigerator at least 8 hours or overnight, turning occasionally.

2 Preheat broiler. Remove beef from marinade; reserve marinade. Thread four (10-inch) skewers with beef, alternating with bell pepper and tomatoes. Spray rimmed baking sheet or broiler pan with nonstick cooking spray. Brush kabobs with marinade; place on baking sheet. Discard remaining marinade. Broil kabobs 3 minutes. Turn over; broil 2 minutes or until desired doneness is reached. Do not overcook. Remove skewers to serving platter.

3 Add remaining 1 tablespoon lemon juice, oil and salt to pan drippings on baking sheet; stir well, scraping bottom of pan with flat spatula. Pour juices over kabobs.

Nutrition Information (per serving)

Calories 193, **Total Fat** 8g, **Saturated Fat** 2g, **Cholesterol** 69mg, **Sodium** 159mg, **Carbohydrates** 5g, **Dietary Fiber** 1g, **Protein** 25g

Dietary Exchanges: 3 Meat • 1 Vegetable

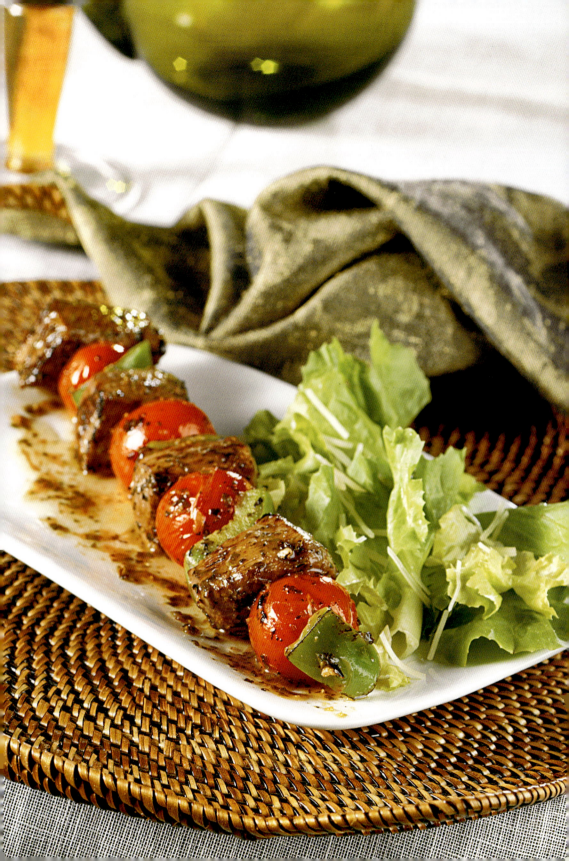

SWEET AND SOUR CHICKEN

Makes 4 servings (¼ of chicken mixture and ½ cup rice per serving)

2   tablespoons unseasoned rice vinegar

2   tablespoons reduced-sodium soy sauce

3   cloves garlic, minced

½   teaspoon minced fresh ginger

¼   teaspoon red pepper flakes (optional)

6   ounces boneless skinless chicken breasts, cut into ½-inch strips

1   teaspoon vegetable oil

3   green onions, cut into 1-inch pieces

1   large green bell pepper, cut into 1-inch pieces

1   tablespoon cornstarch

½   cup fat-free reduced-sodium chicken broth

2   tablespoons apricot fruit spread

1   can (11 ounces) mandarin orange segments, drained

2   cups hot cooked white rice

1 Whisk vinegar, soy sauce, garlic, ginger and red pepper flakes, if desired, in medium bowl until smooth and well blended. Add chicken; toss to coat. Marinate 20 minutes at room temperature.

2 Heat oil in wok or large nonstick skillet over medium heat. Drain chicken; reserve marinade. Add chicken to wok; stir-fry 3 minutes. Stir in green onions and bell pepper.

3 Stir cornstarch into reserved marinade until well blended. Stir broth, fruit spread and marinade mixture into wok. Bring to a boil; cook and stir 2 minutes or until chicken is cooked through and sauce is thickened. Add oranges; cook until heated through. Serve over rice.

Nutrition Information (per serving)

Calories 256, **Total Fat** 2g, **Saturated Fat** 1g, **Cholesterol** 17mg, **Sodium** 320mg, **Carbohydrates** 37g, **Dietary Fiber** 1g, **Protein** 14g

Dietary Exchanges: 2 Bread/Starch • 1 Meat • ½ Fruit • 1 Vegetable

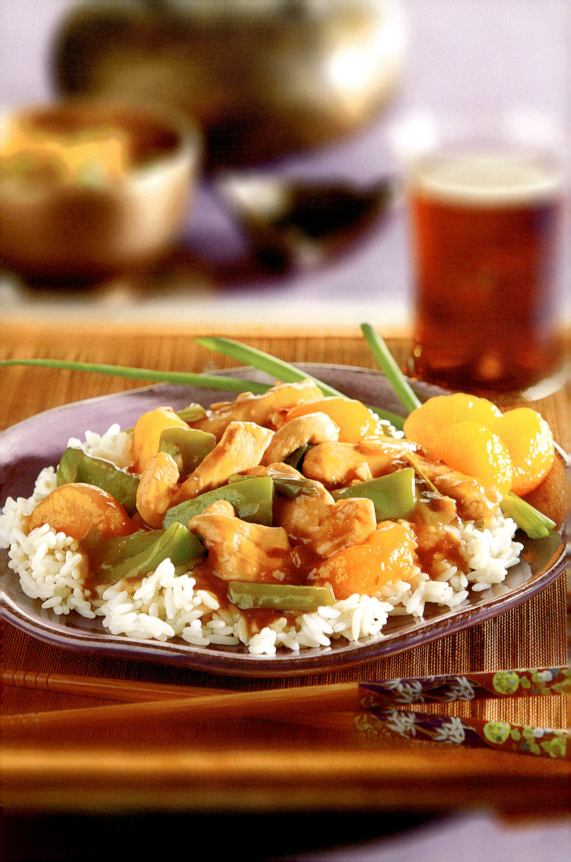

SALMON WITH BROWN RICE AND VEGETABLES

Makes 4 servings (1 cup per serving)

2	cups water
12	ounces skinless salmon fillets
2	cups sliced asparagus (1-inch pieces)
2	cups cooked brown rice
1	cup spinach, sliced into ½-inch strips
⅓	cup fat-free reduced-sodium chicken broth
2	tablespoons chopped fresh chives
2	tablespoons fresh lemon juice
⅛	teaspoon black pepper

1 Bring water to a boil in large skillet over high heat. Add salmon; reduce heat to medium-low. Cover and simmer 10 minutes or until salmon begins to flake when tested with fork. Remove salmon from skillet; cut into large pieces when cool enough to handle.

2 Spray separate large skillet with nonstick cooking spray; heat over medium-high heat. Add asparagus; cook and stir 6 minutes or until tender. Stir in rice, spinach and broth; reduce heat to low. Cover and cook 1 to 2 minutes or until spinach is wilted and rice is heated through. Stir in salmon, chives, lemon juice and pepper.

Nutrition Information (per serving)

Calories 251, **Total Fat** 6g, **Saturated Fat** 1g, **Cholesterol** 47mg, **Sodium** 62mg, **Carbohydrates** 26g, **Dietary Fiber** 4g, **Protein** 22g

Dietary Exchanges: 1½ Bread/Starch • 2 Meat • 1 Vegetable

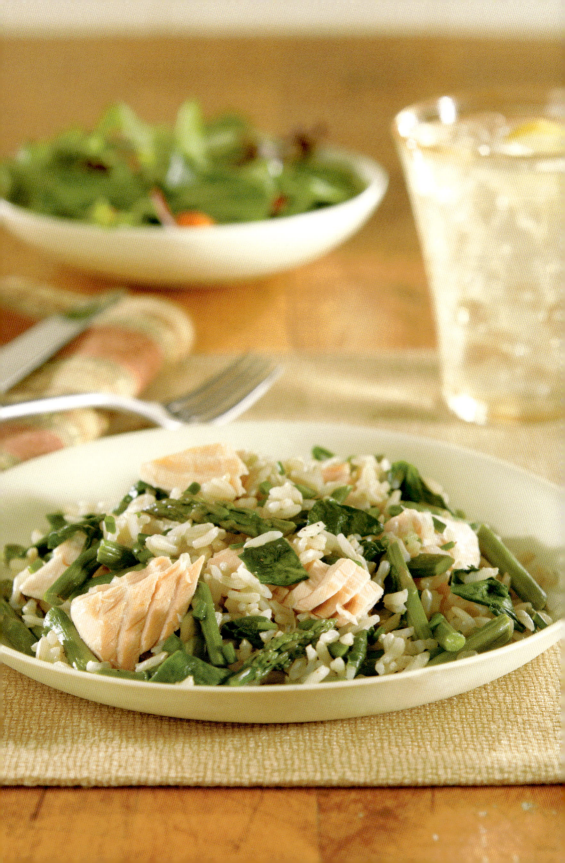

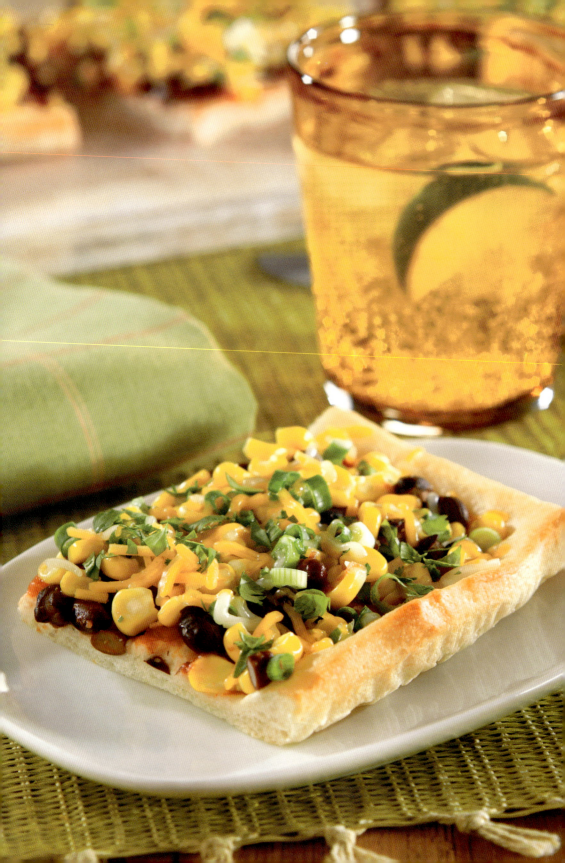

MEXICAN PIZZA

Makes 8 servings

1 package (about 14 ounces) refrigerated pizza dough

1 cup chunky salsa

1 teaspoon ground cumin

1 cup no-salt-added canned black beans, rinsed and drained*

1 cup frozen corn, thawed

½ cup sliced green onions

1½ cups (6 ounces) shredded 2% Mexican cheese blend

½ cup chopped fresh cilantro (optional)

Save the remaining ¾ cup beans (from a 15- or 16-ounce can) in the refrigerator for up to 4 days to add to salads or soups.

1 Preheat oven to 425°F. Unroll pizza dough onto 15×10×1-inch jelly-roll pan coated with nonstick cooking spray; press dough evenly to all edges of pan. Bake 8 minutes.

2 Combine salsa and cumin in small bowl; spread over partially baked crust. Top with beans, corn and green onions. Bake 8 minutes or until crust is deep golden brown. Top with cheese; continue baking 2 minutes or until cheese is melted. Cut into squares; garnish with cilantro, if desired.

Nutrition Information (per serving)

Calories 244, **Total Fat** 6g, **Saturated Fat** 3g, **Cholesterol** 11mg, **Sodium** 699mg, **Carbohydrates** 36g, **Dietary Fiber** 3g, **Protein** 12g

Dietary Exchanges: 2½ Bread/Starch • 1 Meat

COUSCOUS AND VEGETABLE RISOTTO

Makes 4 servings (¾ cup per serving)

- 1 **teaspoon olive oil**
- 1 **rib celery, trimmed and chopped**
- 1 **cup sliced mushrooms**
- 1 **medium yellow or orange bell pepper, cored, seeded and chopped**
- 1 **small onion, chopped**
- 1 **clove garlic, minced**
- ¼ **cup chopped fresh cranberries (optional)**
- ¼ **teaspoon dried crushed thyme**
- ¼ **teaspoon black pepper**
- ⅔ **cup uncooked pearl couscous**
- 1½ **to 1¾ cups reduced-sodium vegetable or chicken broth, divided**
- ¼ **teaspoon salt**

1 Heat oil in large nonstick skillet over medium-high heat. Add celery, mushrooms, bell pepper, onion, garlic, cranberries, if desired, thyme and black pepper. Cook, stirring frequently 6 to 8 minutes or until celery is crisp-tender. Stir in couscous and cook 1 minute, stirring frequently.

2 Pour in ½ cup broth and scrape up browned bits in skillet. Reduce heat to medium-low. Stir in additional ½ cup broth. Cook, stirring occasionally, until broth is absorbed. Add another ½ cup broth. Cook, stirring occasionally. Taste. (Couscous should be tender, but not mushy, and the consistency should be creamy and thick.) If after 15 minutes couscous is still too firm, add remaining ¼ cup broth and repeat cooking and stirring. Stir in salt. Serve immediately.

COUSCOUS AND VEGETABLE SALAD:
Reserve ¾ cup Couscous and Vegetable Risotto; set aside. Combine 1 teaspoon Dijon mustard, 2 teaspoons olive oil, 1 tablespoon white wine vinegar, ¼ teaspoon black pepper, ⅛ teaspoon salt and 1 teaspoon chopped chives in large bowl; mix well. Add 8 ounces bite-sized cooked asparagus, 1 cup cooked chopped chicken breast and reserved Risotto. Mix gently to combine. Makes 2 servings.

Nutrition Information (per serving): Couscous and Vegetable Salad (pictured)

Calories 254, **Total Fat** 8g, **Saturated Fat** 1g, **Cholesterol** 54mg, **Sodium** 433mg, **Carbohydrates** 20g, **Dietary Fiber** 4g, **Protein** 26g

Dietary Exchanges: 1 Bread/Starch • 2 Meat • 1 Vegetable

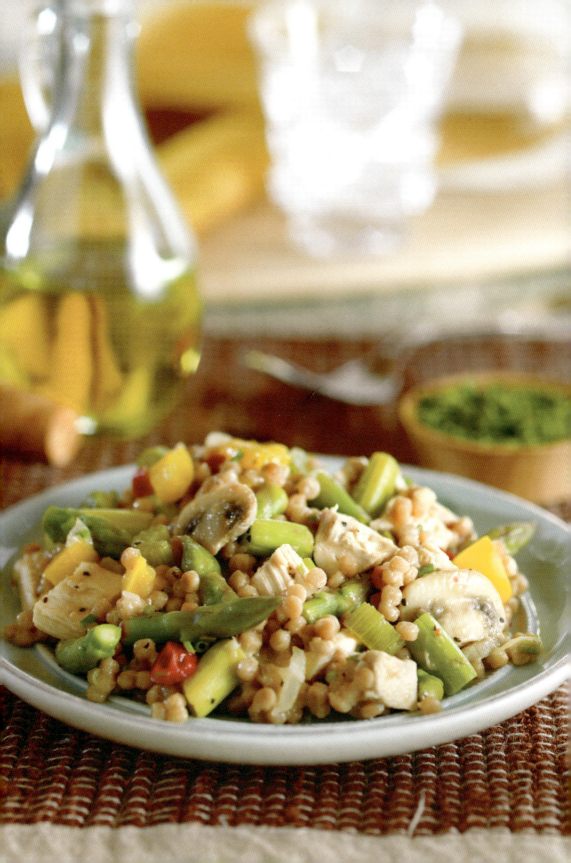

SPROUTS AND BULGUR SANDWICHES

Makes 4 servings (1 sandwich per serving)

½ cup bulgur wheat

1 cup water

1 container (8 ounces) plain low-fat yogurt

¼ cup fat-free salad dressing or mayonnaise

1½ teaspoons curry powder

1 cup shredded carrots

½ cup chopped apple

⅓ cup coarsely chopped peanuts

2 cups fresh alfalfa sprouts

8 very thin slices wheat bread, toasted

1 Rinse bulgur under cold running water; drain. Bring 1 cup water to a boil in small saucepan over high heat. Stir in bulgur. Remove from heat. Let stand, uncovered, 20 minutes. Drain well; squeeze out excess liquid.

2 Combine yogurt, salad dressing and curry powder in medium bowl. Stir in bulgur, carrots, apple and peanuts. Cover and refrigerate.

3 Arrange sprouts on 4 slices wheat toast. Spread with bulgur mixture. Top with remaining bread slices.

Nutrition Information (per serving)

Calories 274, **Total Fat** 9g, **Saturated Fat** 2g, **Cholesterol** 3mg, **Sodium** 439mg, **Carbohydrates** 43g, **Dietary Fiber** 10g, **Protein** 12g

Dietary Exchanges: 2 Bread/Starch • 1 Vegetable • ½ Milk • 1½ Fat

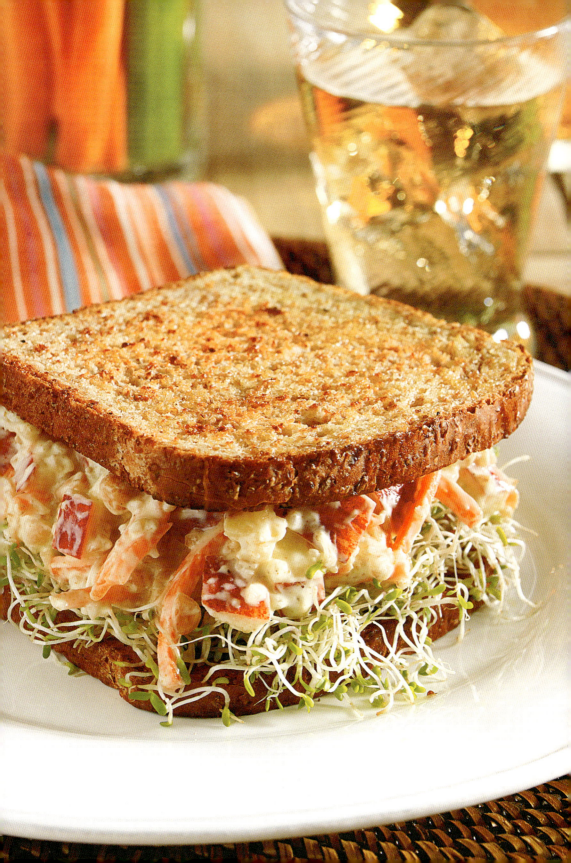

PASTA WITH SPINACH AND RICOTTA

Makes 4 servings (¾ cup per serving)

8 ounces uncooked tri-colored rotini pasta

1 package (10 ounces) frozen chopped spinach, thawed and squeezed dry

2 teaspoons minced garlic

1 cup fat-free or part-skim ricotta cheese

½ cup water

3 tablespoons grated Parmesan cheese, divided

Salt and black pepper

1 Cook pasta according to package directions. Drain well; cover and keep warm.

2 Spray large skillet with nonstick cooking spray; heat over medium-low heat. Add spinach and garlic; cook and stir 5 minutes. Stir in ricotta, water and 1½ tablespoons Parmesan cheese. Season with salt and pepper.

3 Add pasta to skillet; stir until well blended. Sprinkle with remaining 1½ tablespoons Parmesan cheese.

TIP: For a special touch, garnish with fresh basil leaves.

Nutrition Information (per serving)

Calories 286, **Total Fat** 2g, **Saturated Fat** 1g, **Cholesterol** 18mg, **Sodium** 278mg, **Carbohydrates** 48g, **Dietary Fiber** 4g, **Protein** 17g

Dietary Exchanges: 3 Bread/Starch • 1 Meat

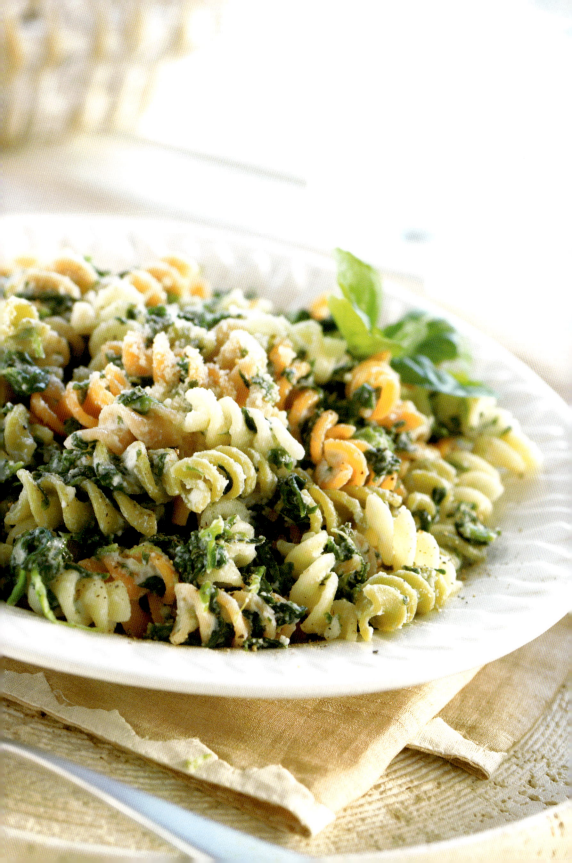

LENTIL BURGERS

Makes 4 servings (1 burger and 1 tablespoon sauce per serving)

1 can (about 14 ounces) fat-free reduced-sodium vegetable or chicken broth

1 cup dried lentils, rinsed and sorted

1 small carrot, grated

¼ cup coarsely chopped mushrooms

1 egg

¼ cup plain dry bread crumbs

3 tablespoons finely chopped onion

2 to 4 cloves garlic, minced

1 teaspoon dried thyme

¼ cup plain fat-free yogurt

¼ cup chopped seeded cucumber

½ teaspoon dried mint

¼ teaspoon dried dill weed

¼ teaspoon black pepper

⅛ teaspoon salt

Dash hot pepper sauce (optional)

Kaiser rolls (optional)

1 Bring broth to a boil in medium saucepan over high heat. Stir in lentils; reduce heat to low. Simmer, covered, about 30 minutes or until lentils are tender and liquid is absorbed. Cool to room temperature.

2 Place lentils, carrot and mushrooms in food processor or blender; process until finely chopped but not smooth. (Some whole lentils should still be visible.) Stir in egg, bread crumbs, onion, garlic and thyme. Refrigerate, covered, 2 to 3 hours.

3 Shape lentil mixture into four (½-inch-thick) patties. Spray large skillet with nonstick cooking spray; heat over medium heat. Cook patties over medium-low heat about 10 minutes or until browned on both sides.

4 Meanwhile, for sauce, combine yogurt, cucumber, mint, dill weed, black pepper, salt and hot pepper sauce, if desired, in small bowl. Serve sauce over burgers.

Nutrition Information (per serving)

Calories 124, **Total Fat** 2g, **Saturated Fat** 1g, **Cholesterol** 54mg, **Sodium** 166mg, **Carbohydrates** 21g, **Dietary Fiber** 1g, **Protein** 9g

Dietary Exchanges: ½ Bread/Starch • ½ Meat • 2½ Vegetable

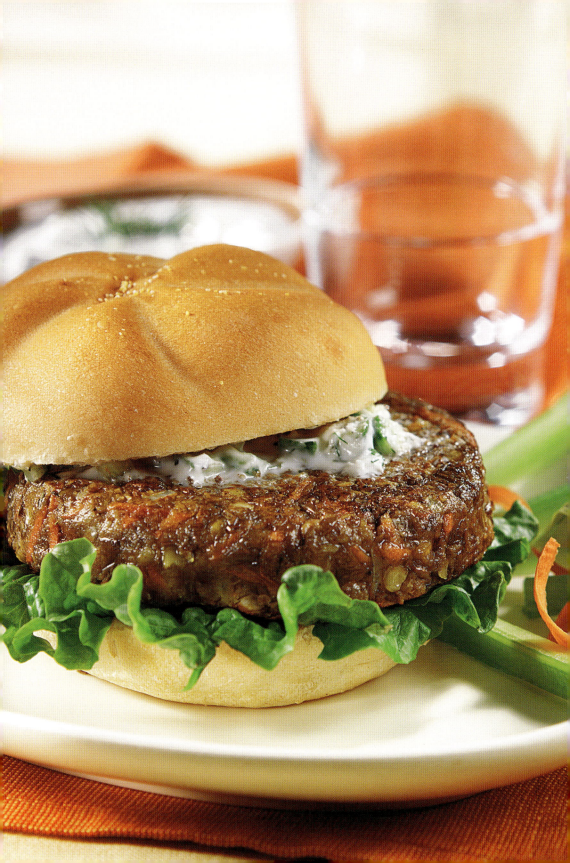

CREAMY SUMMER HERB MAC & CHEESE

Makes 6 servings

3 cups uncooked whole grain elbow macaroni

3 cups finely chopped cauliflower florets

1½ tablespoons blended butter and oil baking sticks

1½ tablespoons all-purpose flour

2 tablespoons minced onion

3 cloves garlic, minced

½ teaspoon salt, divided

1¼ cups fat-free (skim) milk

¼ cup fat-free half-and-half

1 teaspoon chopped fresh thyme, plus additional for garnish

3 light garlic-and-herb spreadable cheese wedges (about 1 ounce each)

2 tablespoons grated Parmesan cheese, divided

1 Cook pasta according to package directions, omitting salt. Add cauliflower during last 5 minutes of cooking time. Drain pasta and cauliflower.

2 Melt butter in medium skillet over medium heat. Stir in flour. Cook and stir 2 minutes or until smooth. Add onion, garlic and ¼ teaspoon salt; cook and stir 1 minute or until onion is softened. Gradually whisk in milk and half-and-half until well blended. Whisk constantly over medium heat 2 to 3 minutes or until sauce boils and is thickened, scraping up brown bits occasionally. Whisk in 1 teaspoon thyme and remaining ¼ teaspoon salt.

3 Remove skillet from heat. Whisk in cheese wedges until cheese is melted and sauce is smooth. Stir in pasta and cauliflower until combined. Gently stir in 1 tablespoon Parmesan cheese.

4 Divide pasta evenly among six serving bowls. Top with remaining 1 tablespoon Parmesan cheese. Garnish with additional thyme.

Nutrition Information (per serving)

Calories 310, **Total Fat** 6g, **Saturated Fat** 2g, **Cholesterol** 5mg, **Sodium** 440mg, **Carbohydrates** 53g, **Dietary Fiber** 1g, **Protein** 14g

Dietary Exchanges: 3 Bread/Starch • ½ Vegetable • ½ Fat

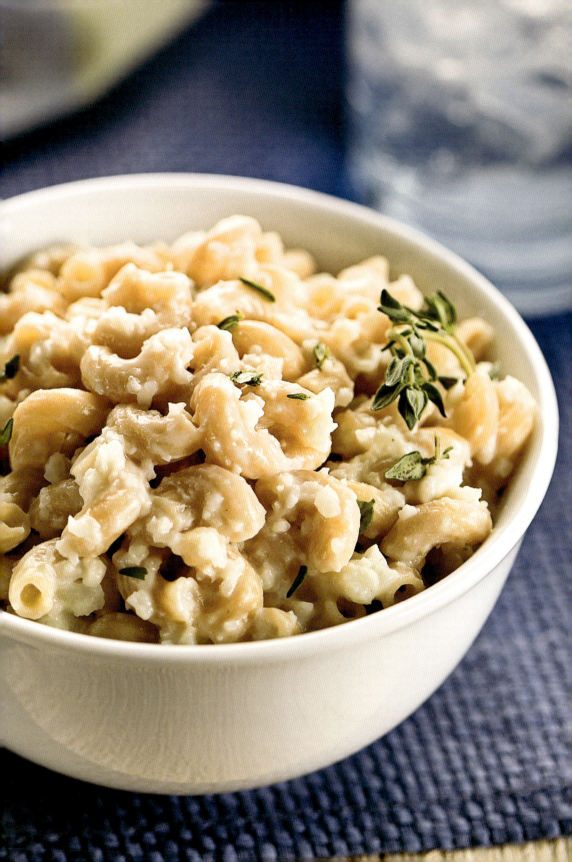

QUINOA BURRITO BOWLS

Makes 4 servings

1   cup uncooked quinoa

2   cups water

2   tablespoons fresh lime juice, divided

¼   cup light sour cream

2   teaspoons vegetable oil

1   small onion, diced

1   red bell pepper, diced

1   clove garlic, minced

½   cup canned black beans, rinsed and drained

½   cup thawed frozen corn

Shredded lettuce

Lime wedges (optional)

1 Place quinoa in fine-mesh strainer; rinse well under cold running water. Bring 2 cups water to a boil in small saucepan; stir in quinoa. Reduce heat to low; cover and simmer 10 to 15 minutes or until quinoa is tender and water is absorbed. Stir in 1 tablespoon lime juice. Cover and keep warm. Combine sour cream and remaining 1 tablespoon lime juice in small bowl; set aside.

2 Meanwhile, heat oil in large skillet over medium heat. Add onion and bell pepper; cook and stir 5 minutes or until softened. Add garlic; cook 1 minute. Add black beans and corn; cook 3 to 5 minutes or until heated through.

3 Divide quinoa among four serving bowls; top with black bean mixture, lettuce and sour cream mixture. Garnish with lime wedges.

Nutrition Information (per serving)

Calories 258, **Total Fat** 7g, **Saturated Fat** 1g, **Cholesterol** 4mg, **Sodium** 136mg, **Carbohydrates** 42g, **Dietary Fiber** 6g, **Protein** 9g

Dietary Exchanges: 3 Bread/Starch • 1 Fat

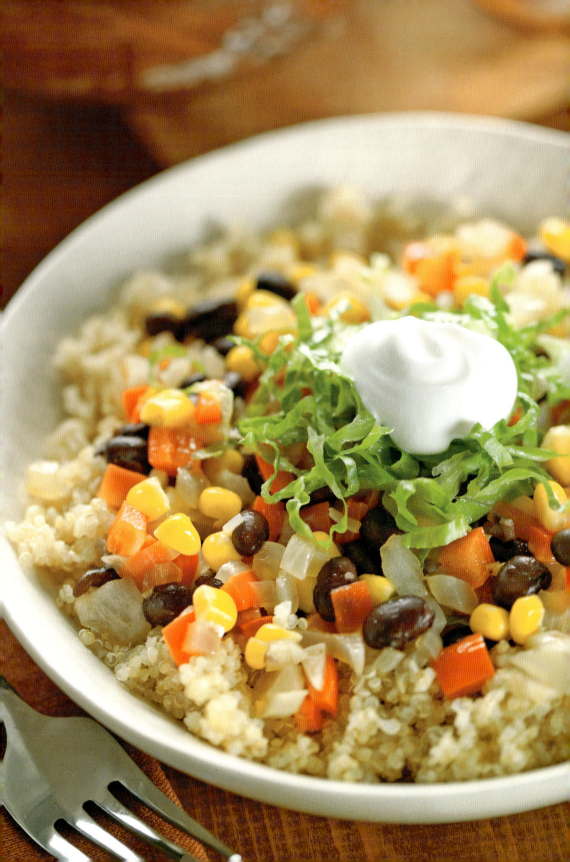

ROASTED EGGPLANT PANINI

Makes 4 servings (1 panini per serving)

1 medium eggplant (about 1¼ pounds)

1 cup (4 ounces) shredded reduced-fat mozzarella cheese

1 tablespoon chopped fresh basil

1 tablespoon fresh lemon juice

⅛ teaspoon salt

8 slices (1 ounce each) whole grain Italian bread

1 Preheat oven to 400°F. Line baking sheet with parchment paper; spray with nonstick cooking spray. Slice eggplant in half lengthwise. Place cut sides down on prepared baking sheet. Roast 45 minutes. Let stand 15 minutes or until cool enough to handle.

2 Meanwhile, combine cheese, basil, lemon juice and salt in small bowl; set aside.

3 Cut each eggplant piece in half. Remove pulp; discard skin. Place one fourth of eggplant on each of 4 bread slices, pressing gently into bread. Top evenly with cheese mixture. Top with remaining bread slices. Spray sandwiches with nonstick cooking spray.

4 Heat large nonstick grill pan or skillet over medium heat. Cook sandwiches 3 to 4 minutes per side, pressing down with spatula until cheese is melted and bread is toasted. (Cover pan during last minute of cooking to melt cheese, if desired.) Serve immediately.

Nutrition Information (per serving)

Calories 310, **Total Fat** 7g, **Saturated Fat** 2g, **Cholesterol** 10mg, **Sodium** 275mg, **Carbohydrates** 50g, **Dietary Fiber** 9g, **Protein** 19g

Dietary Exchanges: 3 Bread/Starch • 2 Meat

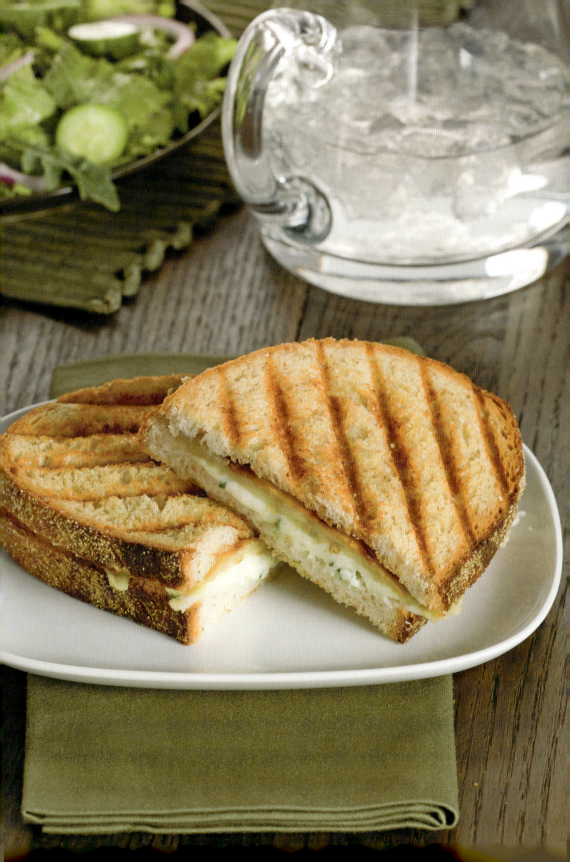

GINGER NOODLES WITH SESAME EGG STRIPS

Makes 4 servings (¾ cup per serving)

5   egg whites

6   teaspoons teriyaki sauce,
　　divided

3   teaspoons sesame seeds,
　　toasted,* divided

1   teaspoon dark sesame oil

½   cup fat-free reduced-sodium
　　vegetable or chicken broth

1   tablespoon minced fresh
　　ginger

6   ounces Chinese rice noodles
　　or vermicelli, cooked and well
　　drained

⅓   cup sliced green onions

*To toast sesame seeds, spread seeds in small
skillet. Shake skillet over medium heat
2 minutes or until seeds begin to pop and turn
golden.

1 Beat egg whites, 2 teaspoons teriyaki sauce and 1 teaspoon sesame seeds in large bowl.

2 Heat oil in large nonstick skillet over medium heat. Pour egg mixture into skillet; cook 1½ to 2 minutes or until bottom is set. Turn over; cook 30 seconds to 1 minute or until cooked through. Gently slide onto plate; cut into ½-inch strips when cool enough to handle.

3 Add broth, ginger and remaining 4 teaspoons teriyaki sauce to skillet. Bring to a boil over high heat; reduce heat to medium. Add noodles; heat through. Add omelet strips and green onions; heat through. Sprinkle with remaining 2 teaspoons sesame seeds just before serving.

Nutrition Information (per serving)

Calories 111, **Total Fat** 2g, **Saturated Fat** 1g, **Cholesterol** 0mg, **Sodium** 226mg, **Carbohydrates** 16g, **Dietary Fiber** 1g, **Protein** 7g

Dietary Exchanges: 1 Bread/Starch • ½ Meat • ½ Fat

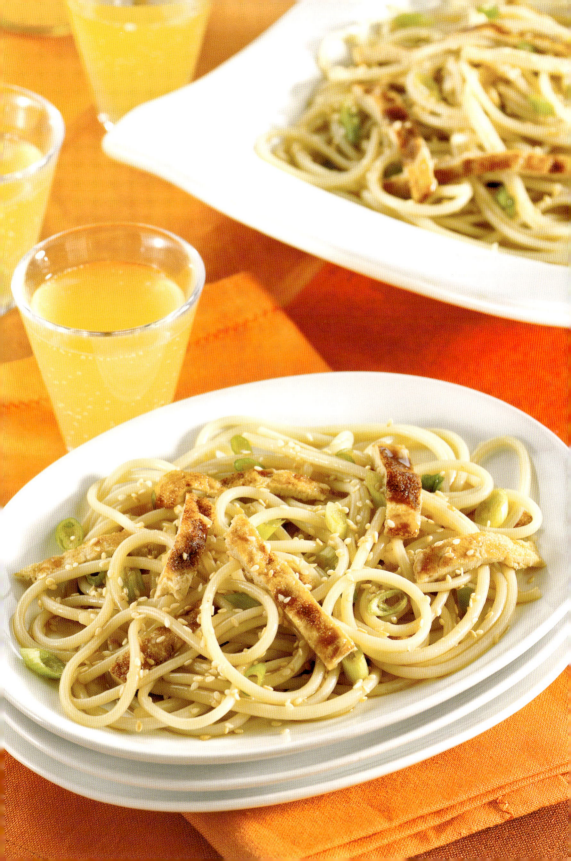

EGGLESS EGG SALAD SANDWICH

Makes 4 servings (1 sandwich per serving)

1 package (14 ounces) firm tofu, drained, pressed* and crumbled

1 stalk celery, finely diced

2 green onions, minced

2 tablespoons minced parsley

¼ cup plus 1 tablespoon vegan mayonnaise

3 tablespoons sweet pickle relish

2 teaspoons fresh lemon juice

1 teaspoon mustard

Black pepper

8 slices whole wheat bread, toasted

1½ cups fresh alfalfa sprouts

8 tomato slices

Cut tofu in half horizontally and place it between layers of paper towels. Place a weighted cutting board on top; let stand 15 to 30 minutes.

1 Combine tofu, celery, green onions and parsley in large bowl. Stir mayonnaise, relish, lemon juice, mustard and pepper in small bowl until well blended. Add to tofu mixture; mix well.

2 Serve salad on toast with alfalfa sprouts and tomato slices.

Nutrition Information (per serving)

Calories 229, **Total Fat** 6g, **Saturated Fat** 1g, **Cholesterol** 0mg, **Sodium** 485mg, **Carbohydrates** 34g, **Dietary Fiber** 5g, **Protein** 13g

Dietary Exchanges: 2½ Bread/Starch • ½ Meat

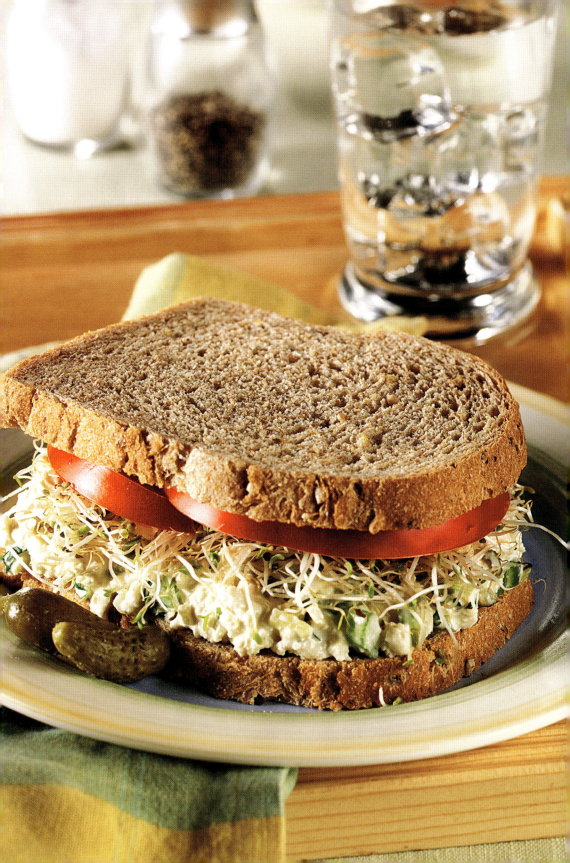

PEPPER PITA PIZZAS

Makes 4 servings (1 pizza per serving)

1 teaspoon olive oil

1 medium onion, thinly sliced

1 medium red bell pepper, cut into thin strips

1 medium green bell pepper, cut into thin strips

4 cloves garlic, minced

2 tablespoons minced fresh basil *or* 2 teaspoons dried basil

1 tablespoon minced fresh oregano *or* 1 teaspoon dried oregano

2 Italian plum tomatoes, coarsely chopped

4 (6-inch) pita bread rounds

1 cup (4 ounces) shredded reduced-fat Monterey Jack cheese

1 Preheat oven to 425°F. Heat oil in medium nonstick skillet over medium heat until hot. Add onion, bell peppers, garlic, basil and oregano. Partially cover; cook 5 minutes or until tender, stirring occasionally. Add tomatoes. Partially cover and cook 3 minutes.

2 Place pita rounds on baking sheet. Divide tomato mixture evenly among pitas; top each pita with ¼ cup cheese. Bake 5 minutes or until cheese is melted.

Nutrition Information (per serving)

Calories 302, **Total Fat** 7g, **Saturated Fat** 3g, **Cholesterol** 20mg, **Sodium** 552mg, **Carbohydrates** 44g, **Dietary Fiber** 2g, **Protein** 16g

Dietary Exchanges: 2 Bread/Starch • 1½ Meat • 2½ Vegetable • ½ Fat

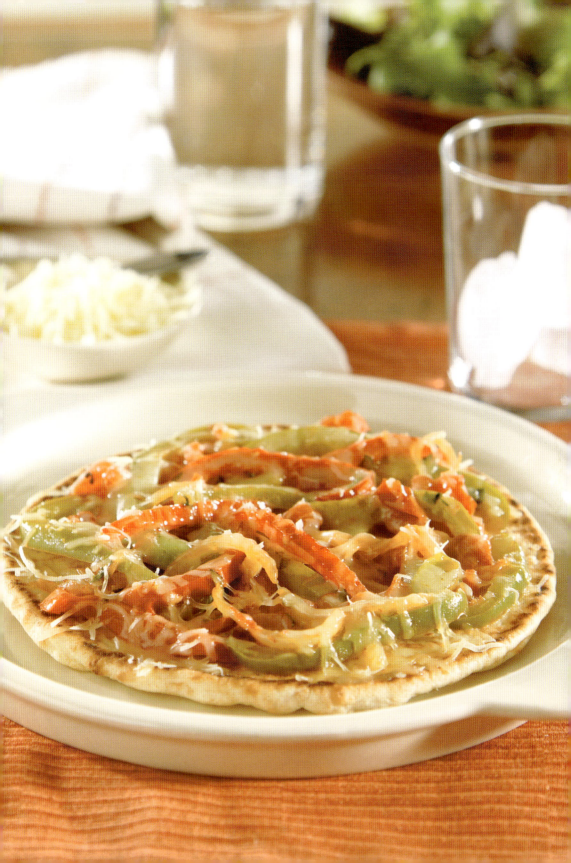

WILD MUSHROOM TOFU BURGERS

Makes 6 servings (1 burger per serving)

3 teaspoons olive oil, divided

1 package (8 ounces) cremini mushrooms, roughly chopped

½ medium onion, roughly chopped

1 clove garlic, minced

7 ounces extra firm lite tofu, crumbled and frozen

1 cup old-fashioned oats

⅓ cup finely chopped walnuts

1 egg

½ teaspoon salt

½ teaspoon onion powder

¼ teaspoon dried thyme

6 light multi-grain English muffins, split and toasted

Lettuce, tomato and red onion slices (optional)

Cucumber spears (optional)

1 Heat 1 teaspoon oil in large nonstick skillet over medium heat. Add mushrooms, onion and garlic; cook and stir 10 minutes or until mushrooms have released most of their juices. Remove from heat; cool slightly.

2 Combine mushroom mixture, tofu, oats, walnuts, egg, salt, onion powder and thyme in food processor or blender; process until combined. (Some tofu pieces may remain). Shape mixture into six (⅓-cup) patties.

3 Heat 1 teaspoon oil in same skillet over medium-low heat. Working in batches, cook patties 5 minutes per side. Repeat with remaining oil and patties.

4 Serve burgers on English muffins with lettuce, tomato and red onion, if desired. Garnish with cucumber spears.

Nutrition Information (per serving)

Calories 254, **Total Fat** 10g, **Saturated Fat** 1g, **Cholesterol** 31mg, **Sodium** 469mg, **Carbohydrates** 37g, **Dietary Fiber** 9g, **Protein** 13g

Dietary Exchanges: 2½ Bread/Starch • 1 Meat • 1 Fat

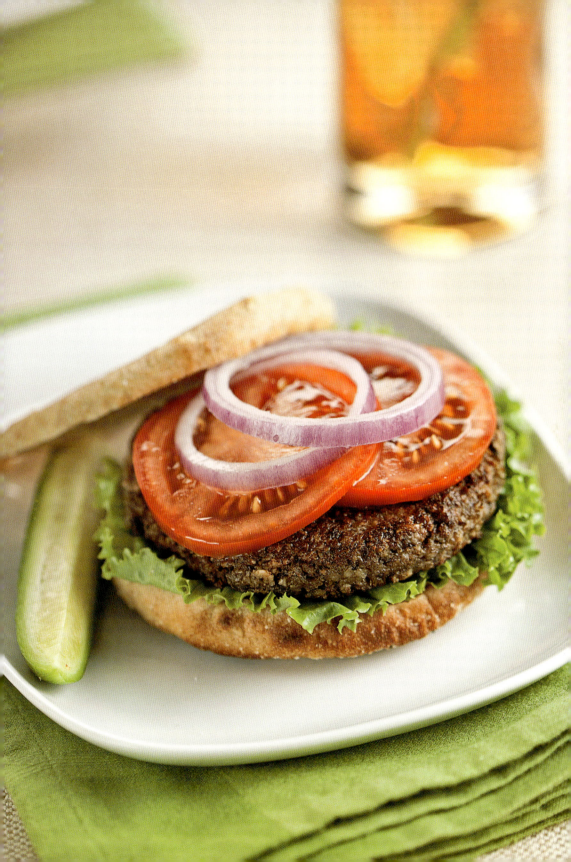

CAVATELLI AND VEGETABLE STIR-FRY

Makes 4 servings (1 cup per serving)

¾ cup uncooked cavatelli or elbow macaroni

6 ounces fresh snow peas, cut lengthwise into halves

½ cup thinly sliced carrot

1 teaspoon minced fresh ginger

½ cup chopped yellow or green bell pepper

½ cup chopped onion

¼ cup chopped fresh parsley

1 tablespoon chopped fresh oregano *or* 1 teaspoon dried oregano, crushed

1 tablespoon reduced-fat margarine

2 tablespoons water

1 tablespoon reduced-sodium soy sauce

1 Prepare cavatelli according to package directions, omitting salt; drain and set aside.

2 Coat wok or large skillet with nonstick cooking spray; heat over medium-high heat. Add snow peas, carrot and ginger; stir-fry 2 minutes over medium-high heat. Add bell pepper, onion, parsley, oregano and margarine. Stir-fry 2 to 3 minutes or until vegetables are crisp-tender. Stir in water and soy sauce. Stir in pasta; heat through.

Nutrition Information (per serving)

Calories 130, **Total Fat** 2g, **Saturated Fat** 1g, **Cholesterol** 0mg, **Sodium** 175mg, **Carbohydrates** 23g, **Dietary Fiber** 3g, **Protein** 5g

Dietary Exchanges: 1 Bread/Starch • 1½ Vegetable • ½ Fat

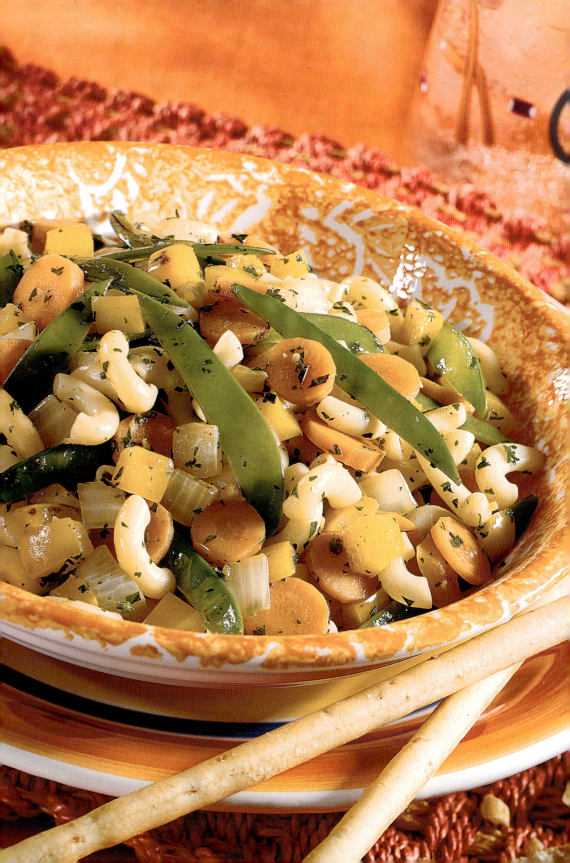

STIR-FRY VEGETABLE PITA PIZZAS

Makes 4 servings (1 pizza per serving)

1 teaspoon olive oil

1 red bell pepper, sliced

1½ cups (4 ounces) baby portobello mushrooms, thinly sliced

1 medium zucchini, thinly sliced

2 cloves garlic, minced

¼ teaspoon black pepper

2 (6-inch) whole wheat pita bread rounds

¼ cup pizza sauce

½ cup (2 ounces) shredded or grated Parmesan cheese

¼ cup chopped fresh basil

1 Preheat broiler. Heat oil in large nonstick skillet over medium-high heat. Add bell pepper; stir-fry 1 minute. Add mushrooms, zucchini and garlic; stir-fry 4 minutes or until vegetables are crisp-tender. Stir in black pepper; remove from heat.

2 Use small knife to cut around edges of pita rounds and split each into two rounds. Place pita rounds on baking sheet. Broil 4 to 5 inches from heat source 1 minute or until lightly toasted. Turn pitas; top with pizza sauce, vegetables and cheese. Return to broiler; broil 3 minutes or until cheese is melted. Top with basil.

TIP: Choose zucchini that are heavy for their size, firm and well shaped. They should have a bright color and be free of cuts and any soft spots. Small zucchini are more tender because they were harvested when young. They should be rinsed well before using, but peeling is not necessary.

Nutrition Information (per serving)

Calories 175, **Total Fat** 5g, **Saturated Fat** 2g, **Cholesterol** 9mg, **Sodium** 381mg, **Carbohydrates** 25g, **Dietary Fiber** 5g, **Protein** 9g

Dietary Exchanges: 1 Bread/Starch • 2 Vegetable • 1 Fat

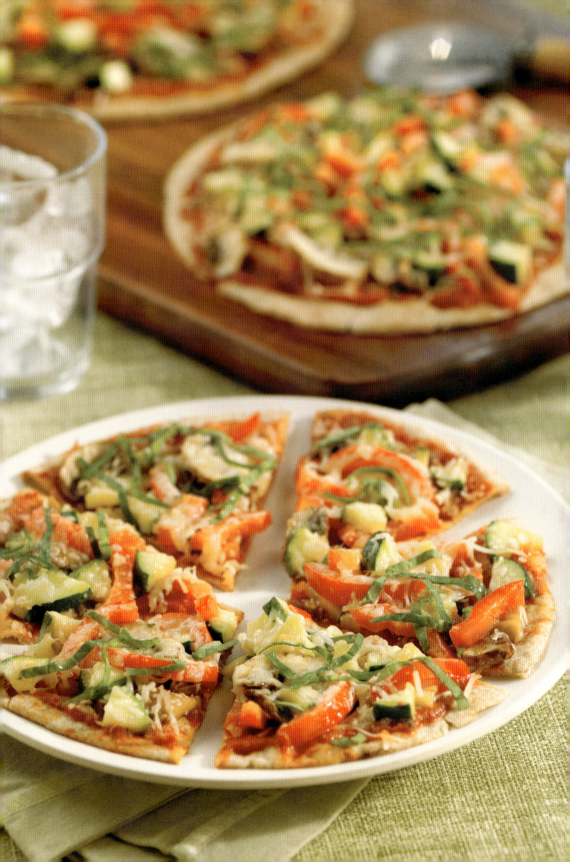

THREE-CHEESE MANICOTTI

Makes 6 servings (1 manicotti per serving)

1 cup sliced cremini mushrooms

2 cups reduced-sodium pasta sauce (without meat)

1 cup fat-free ricotta cheese

¼ cup grated Parmesan cheese

¼ cup cholesterol-free egg substitute

1 tablespoon chopped fresh basil, plus additional for garnish

⅛ teaspoon salt

¼ teaspoon black pepper

6 cooked manicotti shells

¼ cup shredded reduced-fat mozzarella cheese

1 Preheat oven to 350°F. Coat large skillet with nonstick cooking spray. Add mushrooms; cook over medium heat 5 minutes or until tender. Stir in pasta sauce. Spread ½ cup sauce mixture in bottom of 11×7-inch glass baking dish.

2 Combine ricotta cheese, Parmesan cheese, egg substitute, 1 tablespoon basil, salt and pepper in medium bowl. Spoon about ¼ cup mixture evenly into manicotti shells. Place filled shells in baking dish (they should fit snugly). Spoon remaining pasta sauce over manicotti. Cover dish loosely with foil.

3 Bake 28 to 30 minutes or until sauce is bubbly. Remove foil and sprinkle with mozzarella cheese. Bake 5 to 10 minutes or until cheese melts. Let stand 5 minutes before serving. Sprinkle with additional basil, if desired.

Nutrition Information (per serving)

Calories 193, **Total Fat** 6g, **Saturated Fat** 2g, **Cholesterol** 15mg, **Sodium** 263mg, **Carbohydrates** 23g, **Dietary Fiber** 3g, **Protein** 11g

Dietary Exchanges: 1 Bread/Starch • 1 Meat • 1 Vegetable • ½ Fat

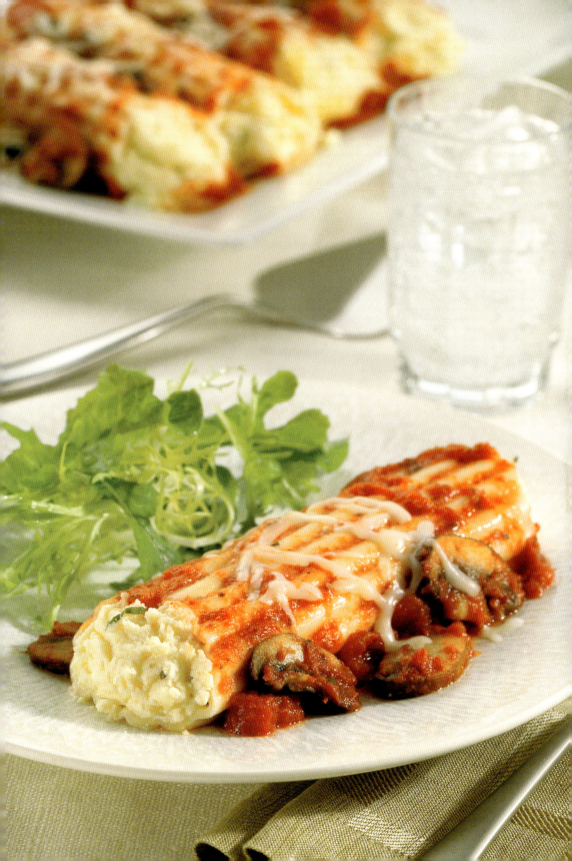

BAKED RISOTTO WITH ASPARAGUS, SPINACH & PARMESAN

Makes 6 servings

1	tablespoon olive oil
1	cup finely chopped onion
1	cup uncooked arborio rice
8	cups (8 to 10 ounces) packed torn stemmed spinach
2	cups vegetable broth
¼	teaspoon salt
¼	teaspoon ground nutmeg
½	cup grated Parmesan cheese, divided
1½	cups sliced asparagus

1 Preheat oven to 400°F. Spray 13×9-inch baking dish with nonstick cooking spray.

2 Heat oil in large skillet over medium-high heat. Add onion; cook and stir 4 minutes or until tender. Add rice; stir to coat with oil.

3 Stir in spinach, a handful at a time, adding more as it wilts. Add broth, salt and nutmeg. Reduce heat and simmer 7 minutes. Stir in ¼ cup cheese. Transfer to prepared baking dish.

4 Bake, covered, 15 minutes. Stir in asparagus; sprinkle with remaining ¼ cup cheese. Cover; bake 15 minutes or until liquid is absorbed.

Nutrition Information (per serving)

Calories 183, **Total Fat** 5g, **Saturated Fat** 2g, **Cholesterol** 7mg, **Sodium** 578mg, **Carbohydrates** 29g, **Dietary Fiber** 2g, **Protein** 7g

Dietary Exchanges: 2 Bread/Starch • 1 Fat

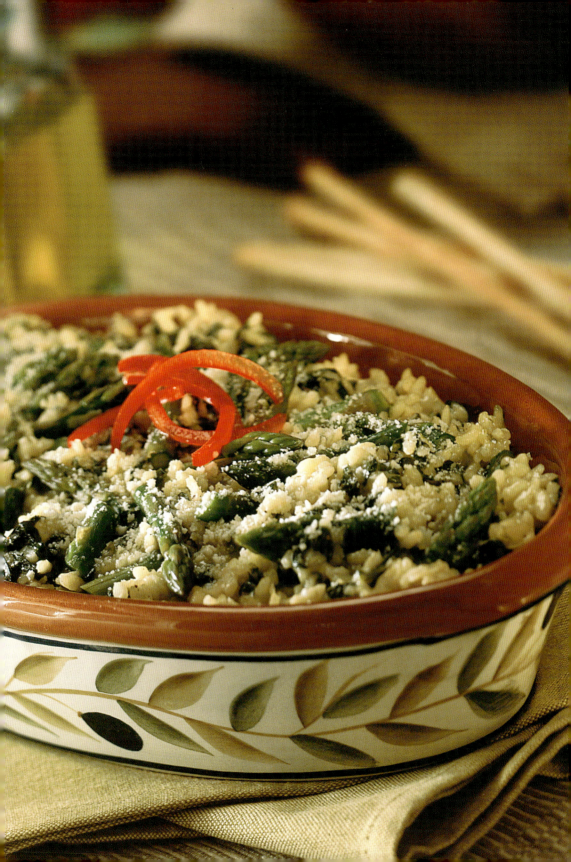

BULGUR PILAF WITH TOMATO AND ZUCCHINI

Makes 8 servings

1   cup uncooked bulgur wheat

1   tablespoon olive oil

¾   cup chopped onion

2   cloves garlic, minced

1   can (about 14 ounces) no-salt-added whole tomatoes, drained and coarsely chopped

½   pound zucchini (2 small), thinly sliced

1   cup fat-free vegetable broth

1   teaspoon dried basil

⅛   teaspoon black pepper

1 Rinse bulgur thoroughly under cold running water, removing any debris. Drain well; set aside.

2 Heat oil in large saucepan over medium heat. Add onion and garlic; cook and stir 3 minutes or until onion is tender. Stir in tomatoes and zucchini; reduce heat to medium-low. Cook, covered, 15 minutes or until zucchini is almost tender, stirring occasionally.

3 Stir bulgur, broth, basil and pepper into vegetable mixture. Bring to a boil over high heat. Cover; remove from heat. Let stand, covered, 10 minutes or until liquid is absorbed. Stir gently before serving.

Nutrition Information (per serving)

Calories 98, **Total Fat** 2g, **Saturated Fat** 1g, **Cholesterol** 0mg, **Sodium** 92mg, **Carbohydrates** 18g, **Dietary Fiber** 5g, **Protein** 3g

Dietary Exchanges: 1 Bread/Starch • ½ Vegetable • ½ Fat

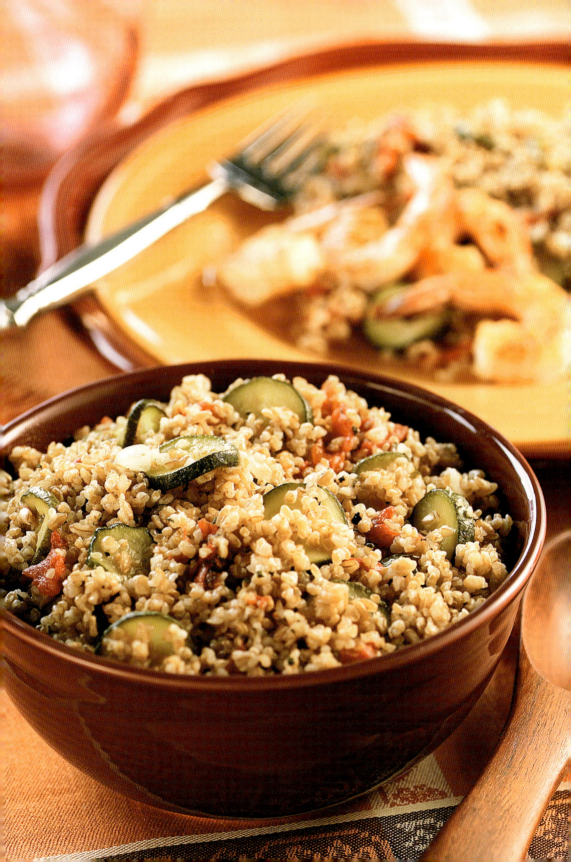

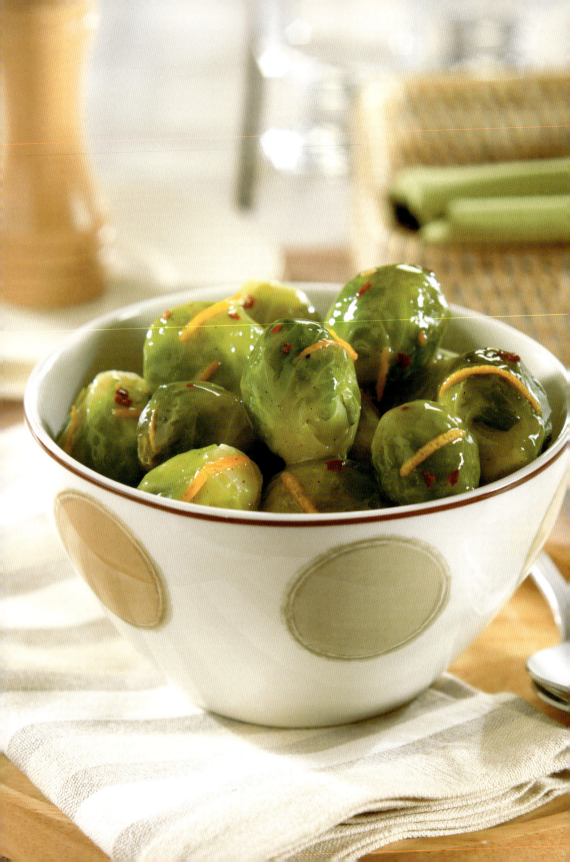

BRUSSELS SPROUTS IN ORANGE SAUCE

Makes 4 servings

4	cups fresh Brussels sprouts
1	cup fresh orange juice
½	cup water
1	teaspoon grated orange peel
½	teaspoon cornstarch
¼	teaspoon red pepper flakes (optional)
¼	teaspoon ground cinnamon
	Salt and black pepper

1 Combine Brussels sprouts, orange juice, water, orange peel, cornstarch, red pepper flakes, if desired, and cinnamon in medium saucepan. Cover and simmer 6 to 7 minutes or until sprouts are nearly tender.

2 Uncover and simmer until most of liquid has evaporated, stirring occasionally. Season with salt and black pepper.

Nutrition Information (per serving)

Calories 59, **Total Fat** 1g, **Saturated Fat** 0g, **Cholesterol** 0mg, **Sodium** 23mg, **Carbohydrates** 13g, **Dietary Fiber** 4g, **Protein** 3g

Dietary Exchanges: ½ Fruit • 1 Vegetable

BUTTERNUT SQUASH OVEN FRIES

Makes 4 servings

½ teaspoon garlic powder

¼ teaspoon salt

¼ teaspoon ground red pepper

1 butternut squash (about 2½ pounds), peeled, seeded and cut into 2-inch-thin slices

2 teaspoons vegetable oil

1 Preheat oven to 425°F. Combine garlic powder, salt and ground red pepper in small bowl; set aside.

2 Place squash on baking sheet. Drizzle with oil and sprinkle with seasoning mix; gently toss to coat. Arrange in single layer.

3 Bake 20 to 25 minutes or until squash just begins to brown, stirring frequently.

4 Preheat broiler. Broil 3 to 5 minutes or until fries are browned and crisp. Spread on paper towels to cool slightly before serving.

Nutrition Information (per serving)

Calories 129, **Total Fat** 3g, **Saturated Fat** 0g, **Cholesterol** 0mg, **Sodium** 155mg, **Carbohydrates** 28g, **Dietary Fiber** 5g, **Protein** 2g

Dietary Exchanges: 1½ Bread/Starch • ½ Fat

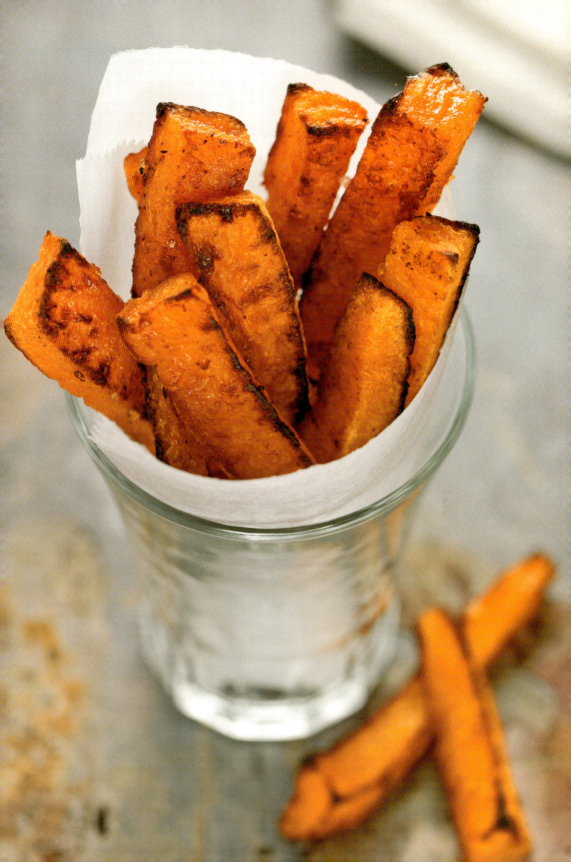

CREAMY COLESLAW

Makes 8 servings (½ cup per serving)

½ cup light mayonnaise

½ cup low-fat buttermilk

2 teaspoons sugar

1 teaspoon celery seed

1 teaspoon fresh lime juice

½ teaspoon chili powder

3 cups shredded coleslaw mix

1 cup shredded carrots

¼ cup finely chopped red onion

Whisk mayonnaise, buttermilk, sugar, celery seed, lime juice and chili powder in large bowl until smooth and well blended. Add coleslaw mix, carrots and onion; toss to coat evenly. Cover and refrigerate at least 2 hours before serving.

Nutrition Information (per serving)

Calories 59, **Total Fat** 4g, **Saturated Fat** 1g, **Cholesterol** 3mg, **Sodium** 143mg, **Carbohydrates** 6g, **Dietary Fiber** 1g, **Protein** 1g

Dietary Exchanges: 1 Vegetable • 1 Fat

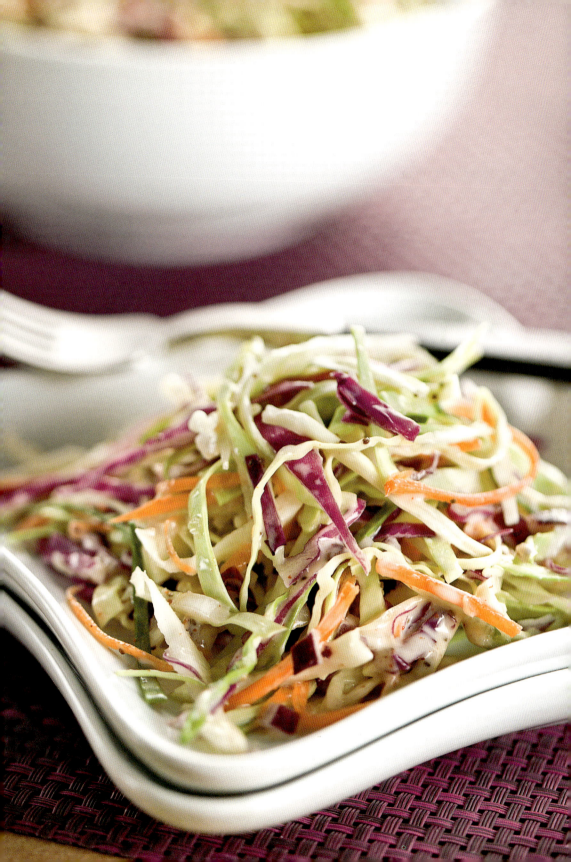

PEPPER AND SQUASH GRATIN

Makes 8 servings

1 russet potato (12 ounces), unpeeled

8 ounces yellow summer squash, thinly sliced

8 ounces zucchini, thinly sliced

2 cups frozen bell pepper stir-fry blend, thawed

1 teaspoon dried oregano

½ teaspoon salt

⅛ teaspoon black pepper (optional)

½ cup grated Parmesan cheese or shredded reduced-fat sharp Cheddar cheese

1 tablespoon butter or margarine, cut into 8 pieces

1 Preheat oven to 375°F. Spray 12×8-inch glass baking dish with nonstick cooking spray. Pierce potato several times with fork. Microwave on HIGH 3 minutes. Cut potato into thin slices.

2 Layer half of potato slices, yellow squash, zucchini, bell pepper stir-fry blend, oregano, salt, black pepper, if desired, and cheese in prepared baking dish. Repeat layers. Dot with butter. Cover tightly with foil; bake 25 minutes or until vegetables are just tender. Remove foil; bake 10 minutes more or until lightly browned.

Nutrition Information (per serving)

Calories 106, **Total Fat** 3g, **Saturated Fat** 2g, **Cholesterol** 8mg, **Sodium** 267mg, **Carbohydrates** 15g, **Dietary Fiber** 2g, **Protein** 4g

Dietary Exchanges: 1 Bread/Starch • ½ Meat • ½ Fat

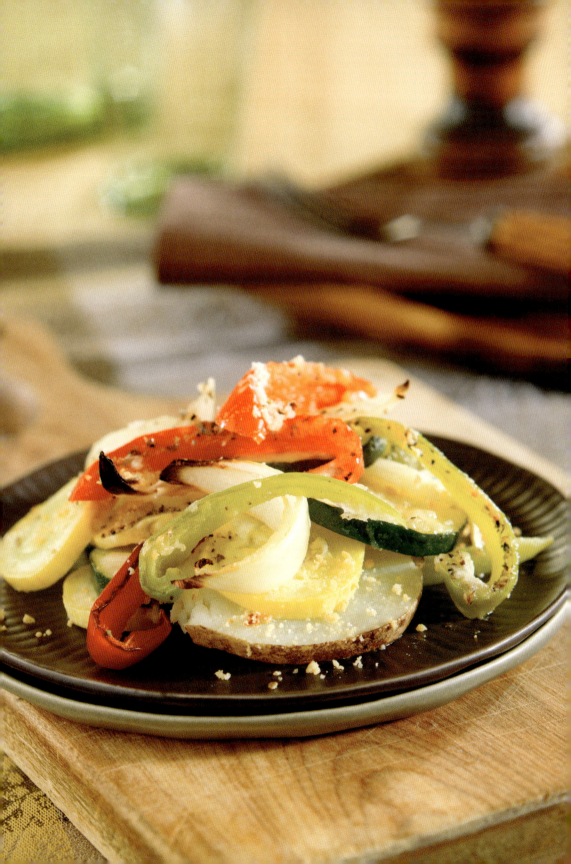

SPICY BAKED SWEET POTATO CHIPS

Makes 4 servings

1	teaspoon sugar
½	teaspoon smoked paprika
¼	teaspoon salt
¼	teaspoon ground red pepper
2	medium sweet potatoes, unpeeled
4	teaspoons vegetable oil

1 Preheat oven to 400°F. Spray baking sheet with nonstick cooking spray. Combine sugar, paprika, salt and ground red pepper in small bowl; set aside.

2 Cut sweet potatoes crosswise into very thin slices, about 1/16 inch thick. Place on prepared baking sheet. Drizzle with oil; toss to coat. Arrange in single layer.

3 Bake 10 minutes. Turn chips over; sprinkle with seasoning mix. Bake 10 to 15 minutes or until chips are lightly browned and crisp, stirring frequently. Spread on paper towels to cool completely.

Nutrition Information (per serving)

Calories 102, **Total Fat** 5g, **Saturated Fat** 1g, **Cholesterol** 0mg, **Sodium** 181mg, **Carbohydrates** 14g, **Dietary Fiber** 2g, **Protein** 1g

Dietary Exchanges: 1 Bread/Starch • 1 Fat

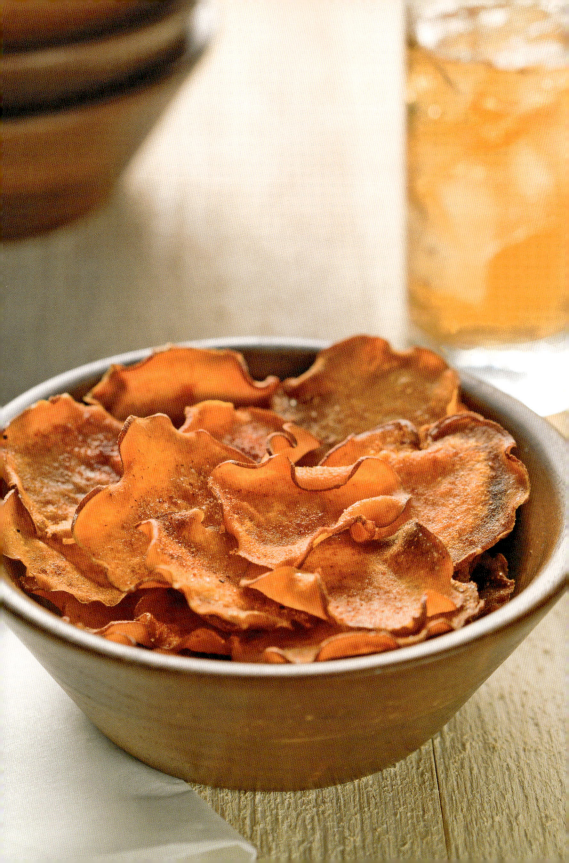

BROCCOLI SUPREME

Makes 7 servings

2 packages (10 ounces each) frozen chopped broccoli

1 cup fat-free reduced-sodium chicken or vegetable broth

2 tablespoons reduced-fat mayonnaise

2 teaspoons dried minced onion (optional)

1 Combine broccoli, broth, mayonnaise and onion, if desired, in large saucepan. Simmer, covered, stirring occasionally, until broccoli is tender.

2 Uncover; continue to simmer, stirring occasionally, until liquid has evaporated.

Nutrition Information (per serving)

Calories 31, **Total Fat** 1g, **Saturated Fat** 1g, **Cholesterol** 1mg, **Sodium** 26mg, **Carbohydrates** 4g, **Dietary Fiber** 2g, **Protein** 2g

Dietary Exchanges: 1 Vegetable

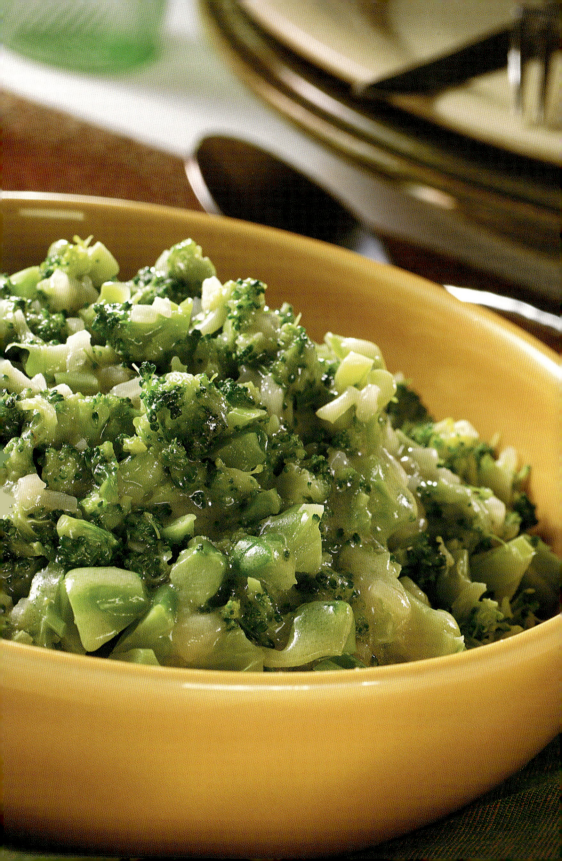

TOFU "FRIED" RICE

Makes 1 serving

2 ounces extra-firm tofu

¼ cup finely chopped broccoli

¼ cup thawed frozen shelled edamame

⅓ cup cooked brown rice

1 tablespoon chopped green onion

½ teaspoon low-sodium soy sauce

⅛ teaspoon garlic powder

⅛ teaspoon sesame oil

⅛ teaspoon sriracha* or hot chili sauce (optional)

Sriracha is a Thai hot sauce that can be found in the ethnic section of major supermarkets or in Asian specialty markets.

MICROWAVE DIRECTIONS

1 Press tofu between paper towels to remove excess water. Cut into ½-inch cubes.

2 Combine tofu, broccoli and edamame in large microwavable mug.

3 Microwave on HIGH 1 minute. Stir in rice, green onion, soy sauce, garlic powder, oil and sriracha, if desired. Microwave 1 minute or until heated through. Stir well before serving.

Nutrition Information (per serving)

Calories 210, **Total Fat** 7g, **Saturated Fat** 1g, **Cholesterol** 0mg, **Sodium** 118mg, **Carbohydrates** 23g, **Dietary Fiber** 5g, **Protein** 14g

Dietary Exchanges: 1 Bread/Starch • 1 Meat • 1 Vegetable • 1 Fat

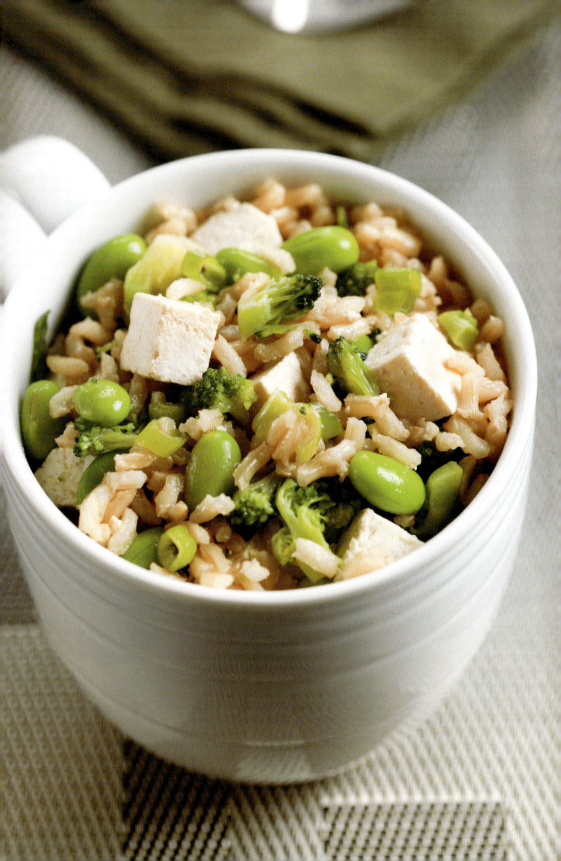

APPLE STUFFED ACORN SQUASH

Makes 8 servings

¼ cup raisins

2 acorn squash (about 4 inches in diameter)

2½ tablespoons margarine, melted, divided

2 tablespoons sugar

¼ teaspoon ground cinnamon

2 medium Fuji apples, cut into ½-inch pieces

1 Cover raisins with warm water and soak 20 minutes. Preheat oven to 375°F.

2 Cut squash into quarters; remove seeds. Place squash on baking sheet; brush with ½ tablespoon margarine. Combine sugar and cinnamon in small bowl; sprinkle half of cinnamon mixture over squash. Bake 10 minutes.

3 Meanwhile, drain raisins. Heat remaining 2 tablespoons margarine in medium saucepan over medium heat. Add apples, raisins and remaining cinnamon mixture; cook and stir 2 minutes. Top partially baked squash with apple mixture. Bake 30 to 35 minutes or until apples and squash are tender. Serve warm.

Nutrition Information (per serving)

Calories 120, **Total Fat** 3.5g, **Saturated Fat** 0.5g, **Cholesterol** 0mg, **Sodium** 35mg, **Carbohydrates** 24g, **Dietary Fiber** 3g, **Protein** 1g

Dietary Exchanges: 1 Bread/Starch • ½ Fruit • ½ Fat

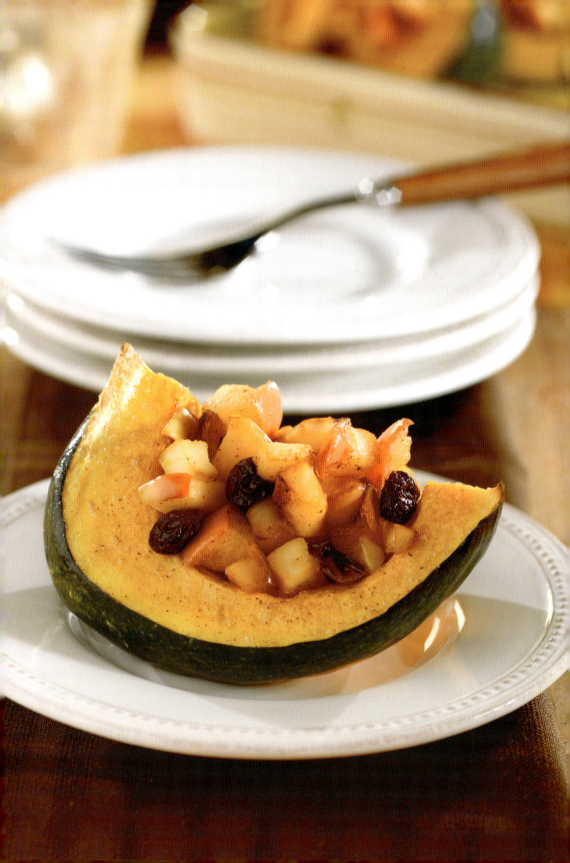

CARAMELIZED BRUSSELS SPROUTS WITH CRANBERRIES

Makes 4 servings (1 cup per serving)

1 tablespoon vegetable oil

1 pound Brussels sprouts, ends trimmed and discarded, thinly sliced

¼ cup dried cranberries

2 teaspoons packed brown sugar

¼ teaspoon salt

Heat oil in large skillet over medium-high heat. Add Brussels sprouts; cook and stir 10 minutes or until crisp-tender and beginning to brown. Add cranberries, brown sugar and salt; cook and stir 5 minutes or until browned.

Nutrition Information (per serving)

Calories 105, **Total Fat** 4g, **Saturated Fat** 1g, **Cholesterol** 0mg, **Sodium** 317mg, **Carbohydrates** 17g, **Dietary Fiber** 4g, **Protein** 3g

Dietary Exchanges: ½ Fruit • 2 Vegetable • ½ Fat

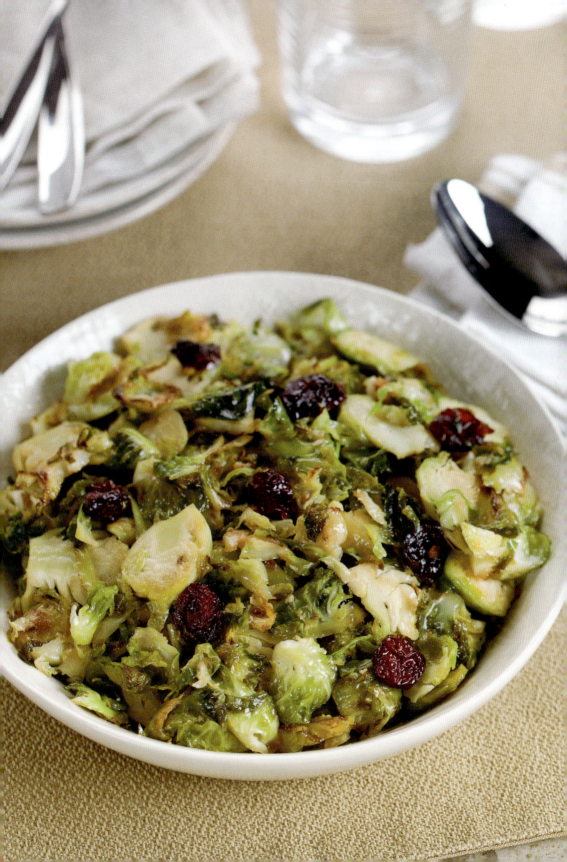

OVEN "FRIES"

Makes 2 servings

2   **small russet potatoes (10 ounces), refrigerated**

2   **teaspoons olive oil**

¼   **teaspoon salt or onion salt**

1 Preheat oven to 450°F. Peel potatoes and cut lengthwise into ¼-inch strips. Place in colander; rinse under cold running water 2 minutes. Drain. Pat dry with paper towels.

2 Place potatoes in small resealable food storage bag. Drizzle with oil. Seal bag; shake to coat evenly. Arrange potatoes in single layer on baking sheet.

3 Bake 20 to 25 minutes or until light brown and crisp. Sprinkle with salt.

NOTE: Refrigerating potatoes—usually not recommended for storage—converts the starch in the potatoes to sugar, which enhances the browning when the potatoes are baked. Do not refrigerate the potatoes longer than 2 days, because they may develop a sweet flavor.

Nutrition Information (per serving)

Calories 237, **Total Fat** 7g, **Saturated Fat** 1g, **Cholesterol** 0mg, **Sodium** 300mg, **Carbohydrates** 41g, **Dietary Fiber** 3g, **Protein** 4g

Dietary Exchanges: 2½ Bread/Starch • 1 Fat

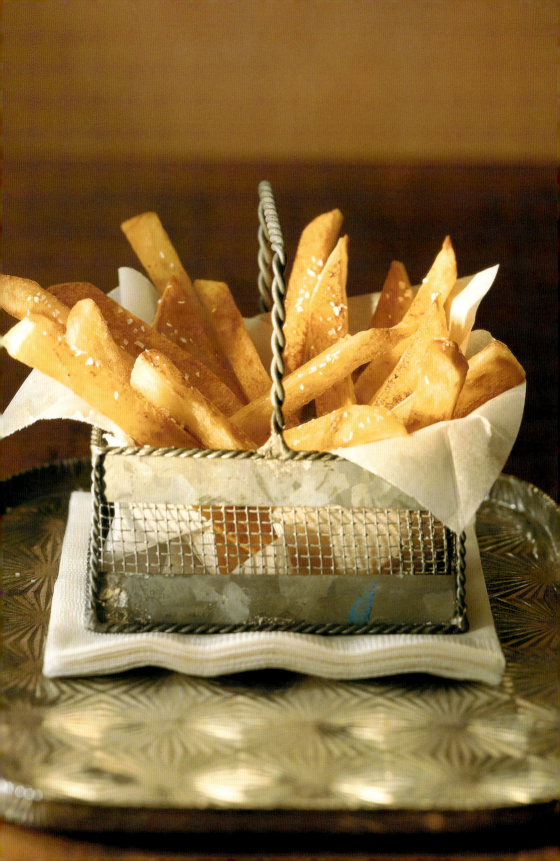

MARINATED VEGETABLES

Makes 12 servings (¾ cup per serving)

¼ cup rice wine vinegar

3 tablespoons reduced-sodium soy sauce

2 tablespoons fresh lemon juice

1 tablespoon vegetable oil

1 clove garlic, minced

1 teaspoon minced fresh ginger

½ teaspoon sugar

2 cups broccoli florets

2 cups cauliflower florets

2 cups diagonally sliced carrots (½-inch pieces)

8 ounces whole fresh mushrooms

1 large red bell pepper, cut into 1-inch pieces

Lettuce leaves

1 Combine vinegar, soy sauce, lemon juice, oil, garlic, ginger and sugar in large bowl. Set aside.

2 To blanch broccoli, cauliflower and carrots, cook 1 minute in enough salted boiling water to cover. Remove and plunge into cold water, then drain immediately. Add to oil mixture in bowl while still warm; toss to coat. Cool to room temperature.

3 Add mushrooms and bell pepper to vegetables in bowl; toss to coat. Cover and marinate in refrigerator at least 4 hours or up to 24 hours. Drain vegetables, reserving marinade.

4 Arrange vegetables on lettuce-lined platter. Serve chilled or at room temperature with toothpicks. Serve remaining marinade in small cup for dipping, if desired.

Nutrition Information (per serving)

Calories 37, **Total Fat** 1g, **Saturated Fat** 1g, **Cholesterol** 0mg, **Sodium** 146mg, **Carbohydrates** 6g, **Dietary Fiber** 2g, **Protein** 2g

Dietary Exchanges: 1 Vegetable

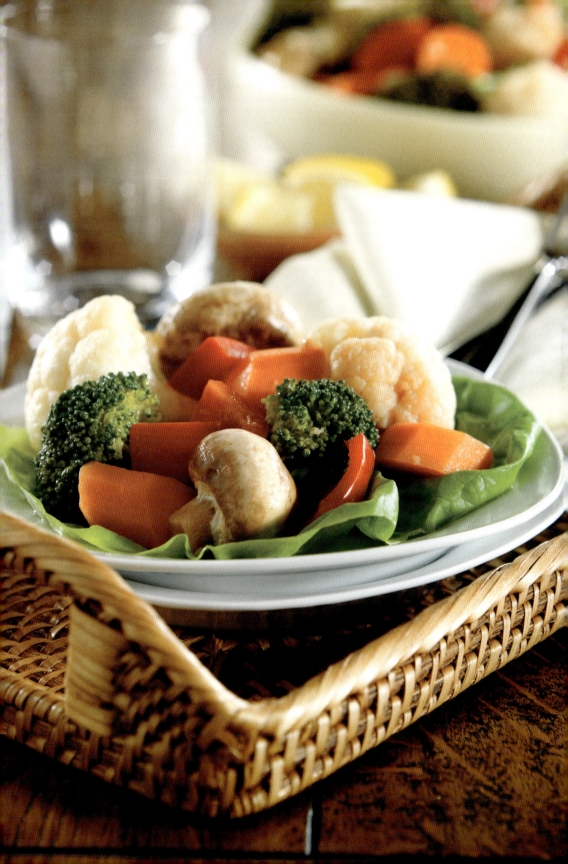

QUINOA & ROASTED VEGETABLES

Makes 6 servings

- 2 medium sweet potatoes, cut into ½-inch-thick slices
- 1 medium eggplant, peeled and cut into ½-inch cubes
- 1 medium tomato, cut into wedges
- 1 large green bell pepper, sliced
- 1 small onion, cut into wedges
- ½ teaspoon salt
- ¼ teaspoon black pepper
- ¼ teaspoon ground red pepper
- 1 cup uncooked quinoa
- 2 cloves garlic, minced
- ½ teaspoon dried thyme
- ¼ teaspoon dried marjoram
- 2 cups water or fat-free reduced-sodium vegetable broth

1 Preheat oven to 450°F. Line large jelly-roll pan with foil; spray with nonstick cooking spray.

2 Combine sweet potatoes, eggplant, tomato, bell pepper and onion on prepared pan; spray lightly with cooking spray. Sprinkle with salt, black pepper and ground red pepper; toss to coat. Spread vegetables in single layer. Roast 20 to 30 minutes or until vegetables are browned and tender.

3 Meanwhile, place quinoa in fine-mesh strainer; rinse well under cold running water. Spray medium saucepan with cooking spray; heat over medium heat. Add garlic, thyme and marjoram; cook and stir 1 to 2 minutes. Add quinoa; cook and stir 2 to 3 minutes. Stir in 2 cups water; bring to a boil over high heat. Reduce heat to low. Simmer, covered, 15 to 20 minutes or until water is absorbed. (Quinoa will appear somewhat translucent.) Transfer quinoa to large bowl; gently stir in roasted vegetables.

Nutrition Information (per serving)

Calories 193, **Total Fat** 2g, **Saturated Fat** 1g, **Cholesterol** 0mg, **Sodium** 194mg, **Carbohydrates** 40g, **Dietary Fiber** 6g, **Protein** 6g

Dietary Exchanges: 2½ Bread/Starch • ½ Vegetable

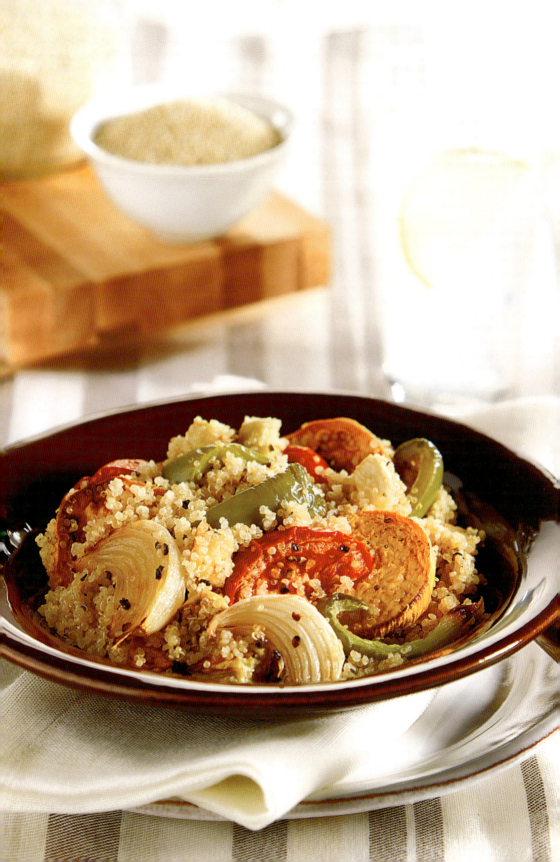

CRUNCHY ASPARAGUS

Makes 4 servings

1 package (10 ounces) frozen asparagus cuts

1 teaspoon lemon juice

3 to 4 drops hot pepper sauce

¼ teaspoon salt (optional)

¼ teaspoon dried basil

⅛ teaspoon black pepper

2 teaspoons sunflower kernels

Lemon slices (optional)

MICROWAVE DIRECTIONS

1 Place asparagus and 2 tablespoons water in 1-quart microwavable casserole dish; cover. Microwave on HIGH 4½ to 5½ minutes or until asparagus is hot, stirring halfway through cooking time to break apart. Drain. Cover; set aside.

2 Combine lemon juice, hot pepper sauce, salt, if desired, basil and pepper in small bowl. Pour mixture over asparagus; toss to coat. Sprinkle with sunflower kernels. Garnish with lemon slices, if desired.

Nutrition Information (per serving)

Calories 29, **Total Fat** 1g, **Saturated Fat** 1g, **Cholesterol** 0mg, **Sodium** 4mg, **Carbohydrates** 4g, **Dietary Fiber** 1g, **Protein** 2g

Dietary Exchanges: 1 Vegetable

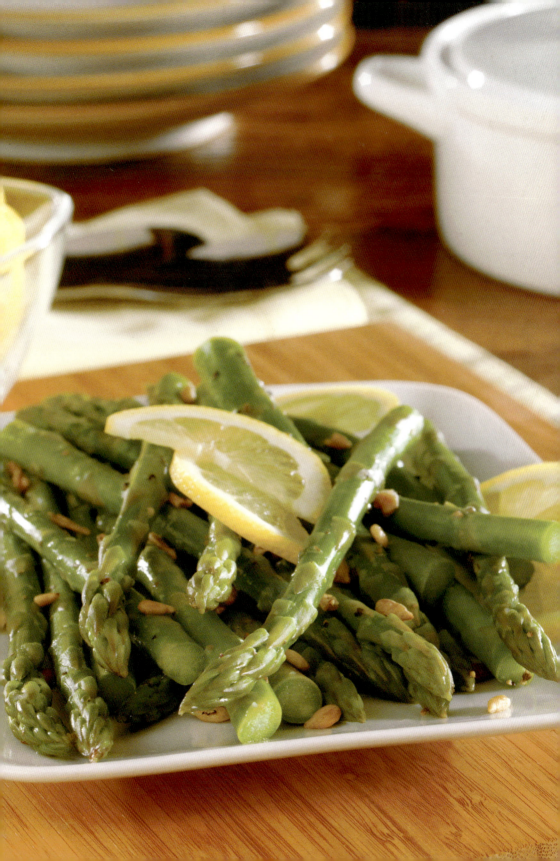

MEDITERRANEAN ORZO AND VEGETABLE PILAF

Makes 6 servings (½ cup per serving)

½ cup plus 2 tablespoons (4 ounces) uncooked orzo pasta

2 teaspoons olive oil

1 small onion, diced

2 cloves garlic, minced

1 small zucchini, diced

½ cup fat-free reduced-sodium chicken broth

1 can (about 14 ounces) artichoke hearts, drained and quartered

1 medium tomato, chopped

½ teaspoon dried oregano

½ teaspoon salt

¼ teaspoon black pepper

½ cup crumbled feta cheese

Sliced black olives (optional)

1 Cook orzo according to package directions, omitting salt and fat. Drain.

2 Heat oil in large nonstick skillet over medium heat. Add onion; cook and stir 5 minutes or until translucent. Add garlic; cook and stir 1 minute. Reduce heat to low. Add zucchini and broth; simmer 5 minutes or until zucchini is crisp-tender.

3 Add cooked orzo, artichokes, tomato, oregano, salt and pepper; cook and stir 1 minute or until heated through. Top with cheese and olives, if desired.

NOTE: This makes a nice side dish to any plain grilled or roasted chicken or fish.

TIP: To reduce the sodium in this recipe, omit the salt. With all the different fresh flavors, you will not miss the extra salt.

Nutrition Information (per serving)

Calories 168, **Total Fat** 7g, **Saturated Fat** 2g, **Cholesterol** 11mg, **Sodium** 516mg, **Carbohydrates** 23g, **Dietary Fiber** 3g, **Protein** 7g

Dietary Exchanges: 1 Bread/Starch • ½ Meat • 1½ Vegetable • 1 Fat

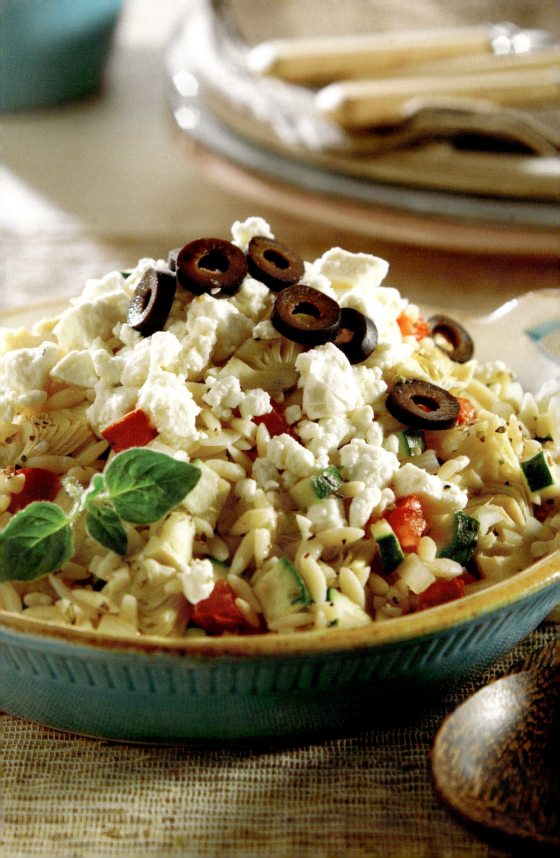

SPINACH CASSEROLE WITH ARTICHOKES

Makes 8 servings (½ cup per serving)

1½ cups diced yellow onions

½ cup fat-free sour cream

⅓ cup reduced-fat mayonnaise

½ cup fat-free (skim) milk

⅓ cup grated Parmesan cheese, divided

2 teaspoons dried oregano

⅛ tablespoon salt

⅛ teaspoon ground red pepper (optional)

2 packages (10 ounces each) frozen spinach, thawed and squeezed dry

1 can (13¾ ounces) quartered artichoke hearts, drained, patted dry and coarsely chopped

1 Preheat oven to 350°F. Coat large nonstick skillet with nonstick cooking spray; heat over medium-high heat. Add onions, coat with cooking spray and cook 4 minutes or until translucent, stirring frequently.

2 Meanwhile, in small bowl, whisk together sour cream, mayonnaise, milk, all but 1 tablespoon Parmesan cheese, oregano, salt and ground red pepper, if desired.

3 Remove skillet from heat, stir sour cream mixture and spinach into onions until well blended. Gently stir in artichokes.

4 Coat 11×7-inch glass baking pan with cooking spray, spoon spinach mixture into pan. Bake, uncovered, 20 to 25 minutes. Remove from oven, sprinkle with remaining 1 tablespoon Parmesan cheese.

Nutrition Information (per serving)

Calories 115, **Total Fat** 4g, **Saturated Fat** 1g, **Cholesterol** 7mg, **Sodium** 517mg, **Carbohydrates** 12g, **Dietary Fiber** 2g, **Protein** 5g

Dietary Exchanges: 2 Vegetable • 1 Fat

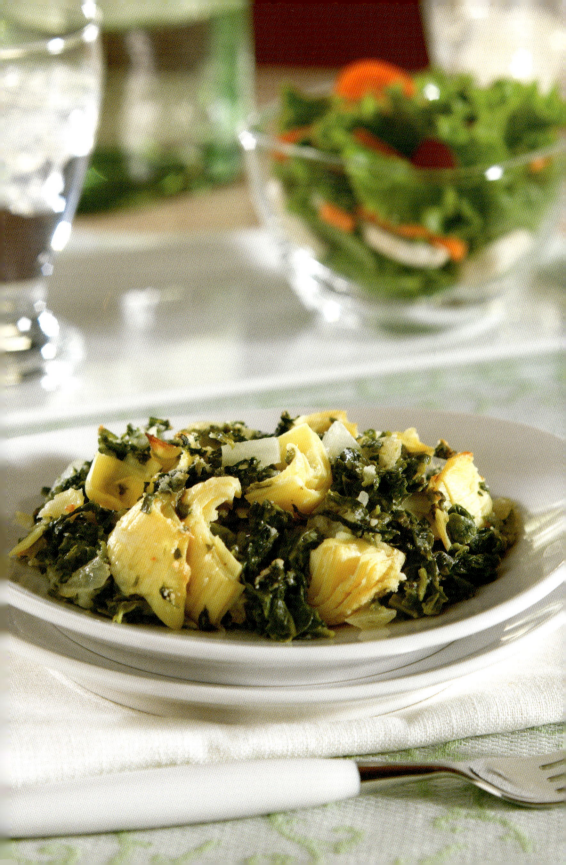

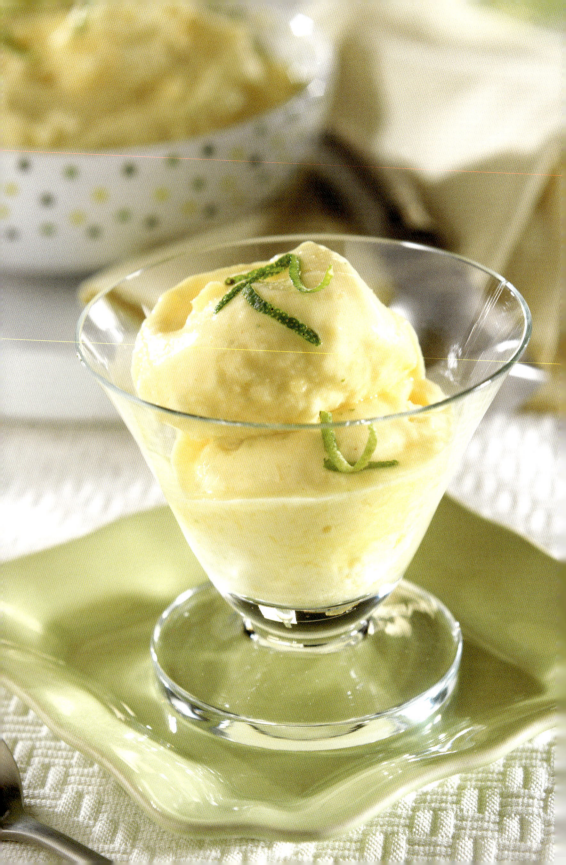

DESSERTS & SWEETS

SPEEDY PINEAPPLE-LIME SORBET

Makes 8 servings (½ cup per serving)

1 ripe pineapple, cut into cubes (about 4 cups)

⅓ cup frozen limeade concentrate

1 to 2 tablespoons fresh lime juice

1 teaspoon grated lime peel

1 Arrange pineapple in single layer on large baking sheet; freeze at least 1 hour or until very firm.*

2 Combine frozen pineapple, limeade concentrate, lime juice and lime peel in food processor or blender; process until smooth and fluffy. If mixture doesn't become smooth and fluffy, let stand 30 minutes to soften slightly; repeat processing. Serve immediately.

Pineapple can be frozen up to 1 month in resealable freezer food storage bags.

NOTE: This dessert is best if served immediately, but it can be made ahead, stored in the freezer and then softened several minutes before serving.

Nutrition Information (per serving)

Calories 56, **Total Fat** 1g, **Saturated Fat** 1g, **Cholesterol** 0mg, **Sodium** 1mg, **Carbohydrates** 15g, **Dietary Fiber** 1g, **Protein** 1g

Dietary Exchanges: 1 Fruit

HIKERS' BAR COOKIES

Makes 24 servings (1 bar per serving)

- ¾ cup all-purpose flour
- ½ cup packed brown sugar
- ½ cup quick oats
- ¼ cup toasted wheat germ
- ¼ cup unsweetened applesauce
- ¼ cup (½ stick) margarine or butter, softened
- ⅛ teaspoon salt
- ½ cup cholesterol-free egg substitute
- ¼ cup raisins
- ¼ cup dried cranberries
- ¼ cup sunflower kernels
- 1 tablespoon grated orange peel
- 1 teaspoon ground cinnamon

1 Preheat oven to 350°F. Lightly coat 13×9-inch baking pan with nonstick cooking spray; set aside.

2 Beat flour, brown sugar, oats, wheat germ, applesauce, margarine and salt in large bowl with electric mixer at medium speed until well blended. Stir in egg substitute, raisins, cranberries, sunflower kernels, orange peel and cinnamon. Spread into pan.

3 Bake 15 minutes or until firm. Cool completely in pan on wire rack. Cut into 24 bars.

Nutrition Information (per serving)

Calories 80, **Total Fat** 3g, **Saturated Fat** 1g, **Cholesterol** 0mg, **Sodium** 46mg, **Carbohydrates** 12g, **Dietary Fiber** 1g, **Protein** 2g

Dietary Exchanges: 1 Bread/Starch • ½ Fat

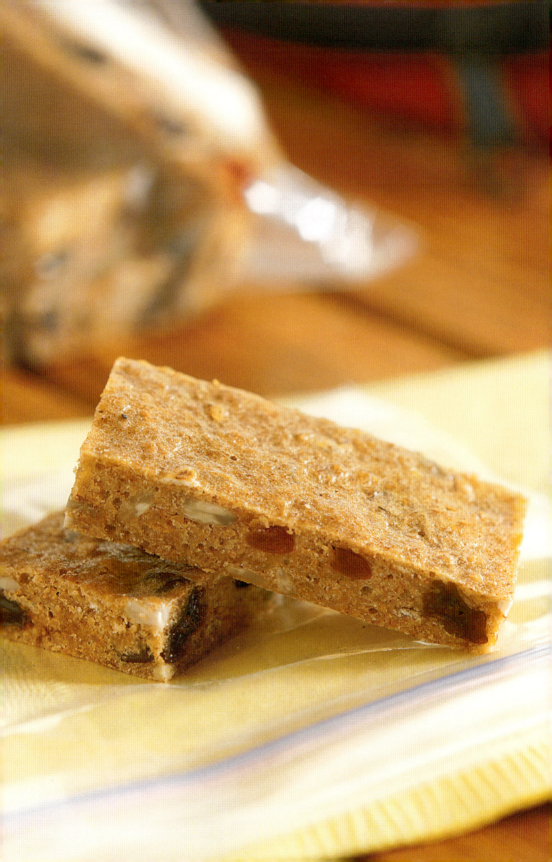

ROCKY ROAD PUDDING

Makes 6 servings (⅓ cup per serving)

5 tablespoons unsweetened cocoa powder

¼ cup granulated sugar

3 tablespoons cornstarch

⅛ teaspoon salt

2½ cups low-fat (1%) milk

2 egg yolks, beaten

2 teaspoons vanilla

6 packets sugar substitute *or* equivalent of ¼ cup sugar

1 cup mini marshmallows

¼ cup chopped walnuts, toasted*

To toast walnuts, spread in single layer in heavy skillet. Cook over medium heat 3 minutes or until nuts are fragrant, stirring frequently.

1 Combine cocoa, granulated sugar, cornstarch and salt in small saucepan; stir until well blended. Stir in milk until smooth. Cook over medium-high heat about 10 minutes or until mixture thickens and begins to boil, stirring constantly.

2 Whisk ½ cup hot milk mixture into beaten egg yolks in small bowl. Pour mixture back into saucepan; cook over medium heat 10 minutes or until mixture reaches 160°F, whisking constantly. Remove from heat; stir in vanilla.

3 Place plastic wrap on surface of pudding. Refrigerate about 20 minutes or until slightly cooled. Stir in sugar substitute. Spoon pudding into six dessert dishes; top with marshmallows and walnuts.

Nutrition Information (per serving)

Calories 190, **Total Fat** 6g, **Saturated Fat** 1g, **Cholesterol** 75mg, **Sodium** 121mg, **Carbohydrates** 28g, **Dietary Fiber** 1g, **Protein** 7g

Dietary Exchanges: 1 Bread/Starch • ½ Milk • 1 Fat

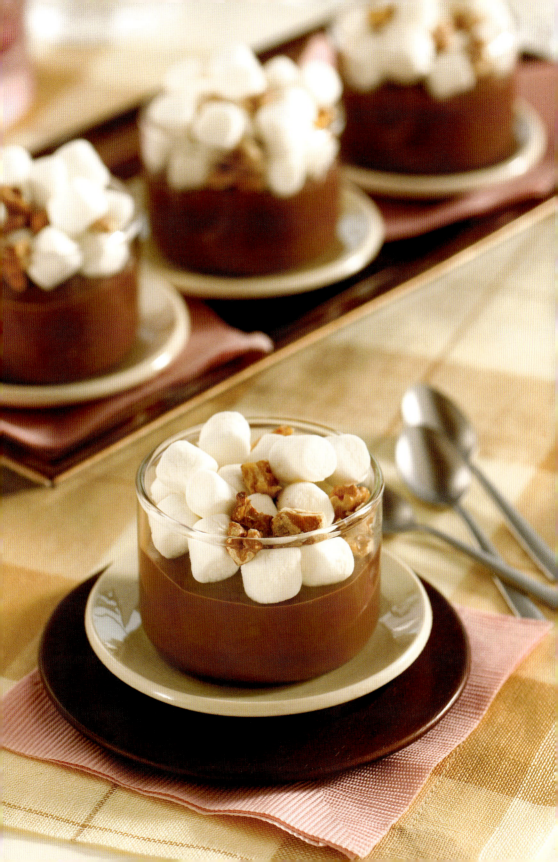

FRUIT SALAD WITH CREAMY BANANA DRESSING

Makes 8 servings

2 cups fresh pineapple chunks

1 cup cantaloupe cubes

1 cup honeydew melon cubes

1 cup fresh blackberries

1 cup sliced fresh strawberries

1 cup seedless red grapes

1 medium apple, diced

2 medium ripe bananas, sliced

½ cup vanilla nonfat Greek yogurt

2 tablespoons honey

1 tablespoon fresh lemon juice

¼ teaspoon ground nutmeg

1 Combine pineapple, cantaloupe, honeydew, blackberries, strawberries, grapes and apple in large bowl; gently mix.

2 Combine bananas, yogurt, honey, lemon juice and nutmeg in blender or food processor; blend until smooth.

3 Pour dressing over fruit mixture; gently toss to coat evenly. Serve immediately.

Nutrition Information (per serving)

Calories 125, **Total Fat** 0g, **Saturated Fat** 0g, **Cholesterol** 0mg, **Sodium** 15mg, **Carbohydrates** 31g, **Dietary Fiber** 4g, **Protein** 3g

Dietary Exchanges: 2 Fruit

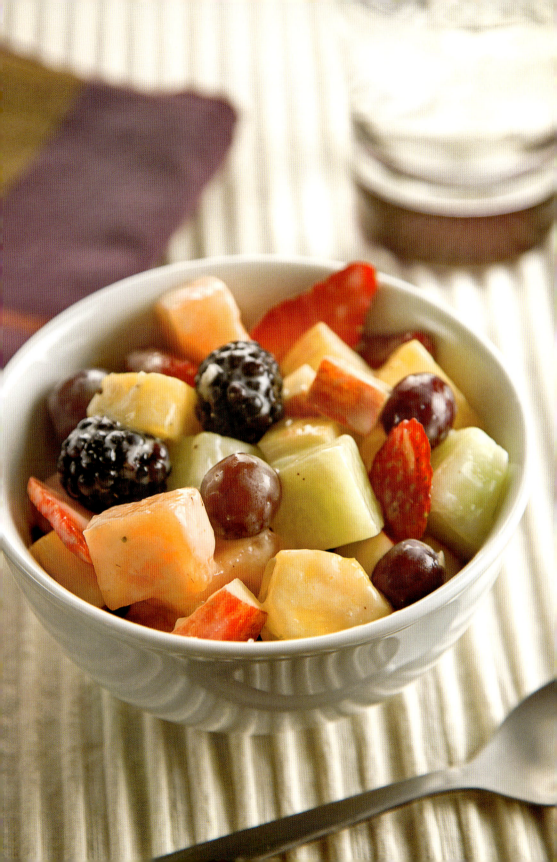

MOCHA CRINKLES

Makes about 6 dozen cookies (1 cookie per serving)

1⅓	**cups packed light brown sugar**
½	**cup vegetable oil**
¼	**cup light sour cream**
1	**egg**
1	**teaspoon vanilla**
1¾	**cups all-purpose flour**
¾	**cup unsweetened cocoa powder**
2	**teaspoons instant coffee granules**
1	**teaspoon baking soda**
¼	**teaspoon salt**
⅛	**teaspoon black pepper**
½	**cup powdered sugar**

1 Beat brown sugar and oil in large bowl with electric mixer at medium speed until well blended. Add sour cream, egg and vanilla; beat until well blended. Combine flour, cocoa, coffee granules, baking soda, salt and pepper in medium bowl; mix well. Beat into brown sugar mixture until well blended. Cover and refrigerate 3 to 4 hours.

2 Preheat oven to 350°F. Place powdered sugar in shallow bowl. Shape dough into 1-inch balls; roll in powdered sugar. Place 2 inches apart on ungreased cookie sheets.

3 Bake 10 to 12 minutes or until tops of cookies are firm. *Do not overbake.* Remove to wire racks; cool completely.

Nutrition Information (per serving)

Calories 44, **Total Fat** 1g, **Saturated Fat** 1g, **Cholesterol** 3mg, **Sodium** 28mg, **Carbohydrates** 7g, **Dietary Fiber** 0g, **Protein** 0g

Dietary Exchanges: ½ Bread/Starch

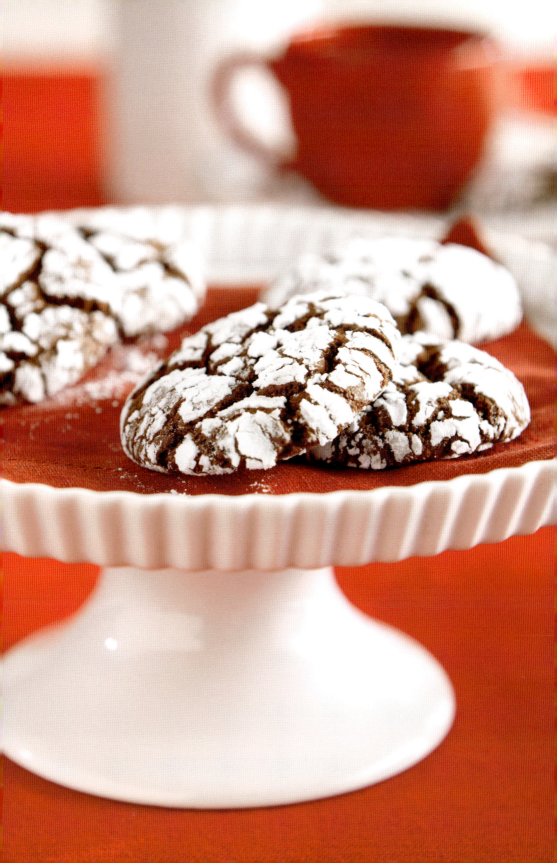

WATERMELON ICE

Makes 6 servings (½ cup per serving)

4   cups seeded 1-inch watermelon chunks

¼   cup thawed frozen unsweetened pineapple juice concentrate

2   tablespoons fresh lime juice

Fresh melon balls (optional)

Fresh mint leaves (optional)

1 Place melon chunks in single layer in large resealable freezer food storage bag; freeze 8 hours or until firm.

2 Place frozen melon in food processor container fitted with steel blade. Let stand 15 to 20 minutes to soften slightly. Add pineapple juice concentrate and lime juice. Remove plunger from top of food processor to allow air to be incorporated. Process until smooth, scraping down sides of container frequently.

3 Spoon into individual dessert dishes. Garnish with melon balls and mint leaves, if desired. Serve immediately.

HONEYDEW ICE: Substitute honeydew for watermelon and unsweetened pineapple-guava-orange juice concentrate for pineapple juice concentrate.

CANTALOUPE ICE: Substitute cantaloupe for watermelon and unsweetened pineapple-guava-orange juice concentrate for pineapple juice concentrate.

NOTE: Ices can be transferred to airtight container and frozen up to 1 month. Let stand at room temperature 10 minutes to soften slightly before serving.

Nutrition Information (per serving)

Calories 57, **Total Fat** 1g, **Saturated Fat** 1g, **Cholesterol** 0mg, **Sodium** 3mg, **Carbohydrates** 13g, **Dietary Fiber** 1g, **Protein** 1g

Dietary Exchanges: 1 Fruit

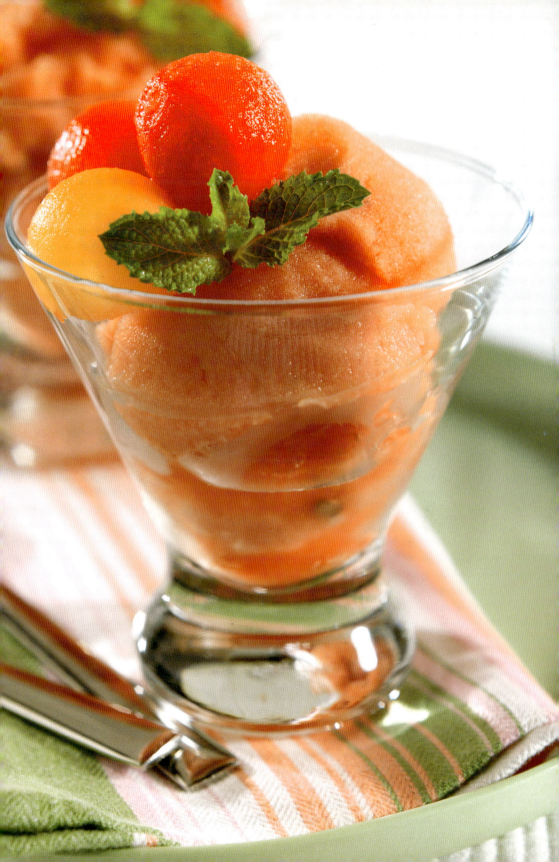

PEACH-MELBA SHORTCAKES

Makes 4 servings

1 cup reduced-fat biscuit baking mix

¼ cup fat-free (skim) milk

2 tablespoons sugar

1¼ cups fresh raspberries

1 cup diced peeled peaches

2 tablespoons raspberry fruit spread

4 tablespoons thawed frozen whipped topping

1 Preheat oven to 425°F. Stir baking mix, milk and sugar in small bowl until smooth and well blended. Drop about 3 tablespoons per biscuit onto ungreased baking sheet. Bake 10 to 12 minutes or until tops are slightly browned. Cool on baking sheet 5 minutes.

2 Meanwhile, combine raspberries and peaches in medium bowl; set aside.

3 Microwave fruit spread in small microwavable bowl on HIGH 15 seconds or until softened.

4 Slice warm biscuits in half. Arrange biscuit bottoms on four serving plates. Drizzle ½ teaspoon fruit spread over each biscuit bottom. Top evenly with raspberries and peaches. Replace biscuit tops. Drizzle each shortcake with 1 teaspoon fruit spread; top with 1 tablespoon whipped topping.

Nutrition Information (per serving)

Calories 205, **Total Fat** 3g, **Saturated Fat** 1g, **Cholesterol** 0mg, **Sodium** 335mg, **Carbohydrates** 42g, **Dietary Fiber** 4g, **Protein** 4g

Dietary Exchanges: 2 Bread/Starch • 1 Fruit

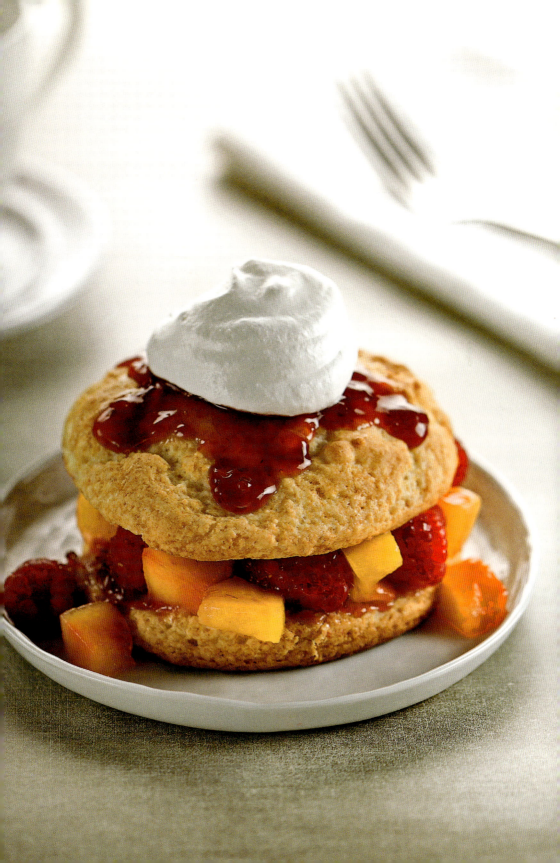

PUMPKIN CAKE WITH CREAMY ORANGE GLAZE

Makes 24 servings

CAKE

2	cups all-purpose flour
2	teaspoons baking powder
2	teaspoons ground cinnamon
1	teaspoon baking soda
1	teaspoon salt
1	teaspoon ground ginger
1	teaspoon ground nutmeg
1	can (15 ounces) solid-pack pumpkin
3	eggs
¾	cup packed brown sugar
½	cup granulated sugar
½	cup natural or unsweetened applesauce
2	tablespoons vegetable oil

GLAZE

2	ounces light cream cheese, softened
¼	cup powdered sugar
2	to 4 tablespoons fat-free (skim) milk
¼	teaspoon orange extract

1 Preheat the oven to 350°F. Spray 13×9-inch baking pan with nonstick cooking spray.

2 Combine flour, baking powder, cinnamon, baking soda, salt, ginger and nutmeg in medium bowl; mix well. Stir pumpkin, eggs, brown sugar, granulated sugar, applesauce and oil in large bowl until smooth and well blended. Gradually stir in flour mixture until smooth and well blended. Pour into prepared pan.

3 Bake 30 to 35 minutes or until toothpick inserted into center comes out clean. Cool completely in pan on wire rack.

4 Beat cream cheese in medium bowl until smooth. Add powdered sugar; beat until well blended. Add 2 tablespoons milk and orange extract; beat until smooth. Add additional milk, 1 teaspoon at a time, until desired consistency is reached.

5 Spread glaze over cake. Let stand until set before cutting and serving.

Nutrition Information (per serving)

Calories 120, **Total Fat** 2g, **Saturated Fat** 1g, **Cholesterol** 25mg, **Sodium** 213mg, **Carbohydrates** 23g, **Dietary Fiber** 1g, **Protein** 2g

Dietary Exchanges: 1 Bread/Starch • ½ Fruit • ½ Fat

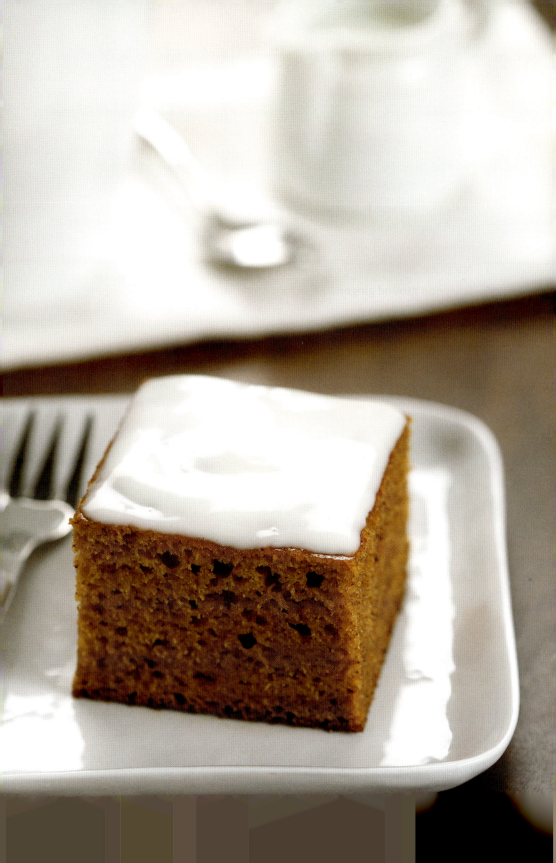

MINI LEMON CHEESECAKES

Makes 12 servings

1 package (8 ounces) light cream cheese, softened

1 package (8 ounces) fat-free cream cheese, softened

2 eggs

½ cup sugar

Grated peel of 1 lemon, plus additional for garnish

Juice of 1 lemon

1 Preheat oven to 325°F. Line 12 standard (2½-inch) muffin cups with foil baking cups; spray with nonstick cooking spray.

2 Beat cream cheeses, eggs, sugar, grated peel of 1 lemon and lemon juice in medium bowl with electric mixer at medium speed until smooth and well blended. Spoon evenly into prepared muffin cups.

3 Bake 25 to 30 minutes or until almost set. (Centers will be spongy to the touch). Cool in pans 10 minutes. Refrigerate at least 1 hour before serving. Garnish with additional lemon peel.

Nutrition Information (per serving)

Calories 104, **Total Fat** 4g, **Saturated Fat** 2g, **Cholesterol** 44mg, **Sodium** 234mg, **Carbohydrates** 12g, **Dietary Fiber** 0g, **Protein** 6g

Dietary Exchanges: 1 Bread/Starch • ½ Fat

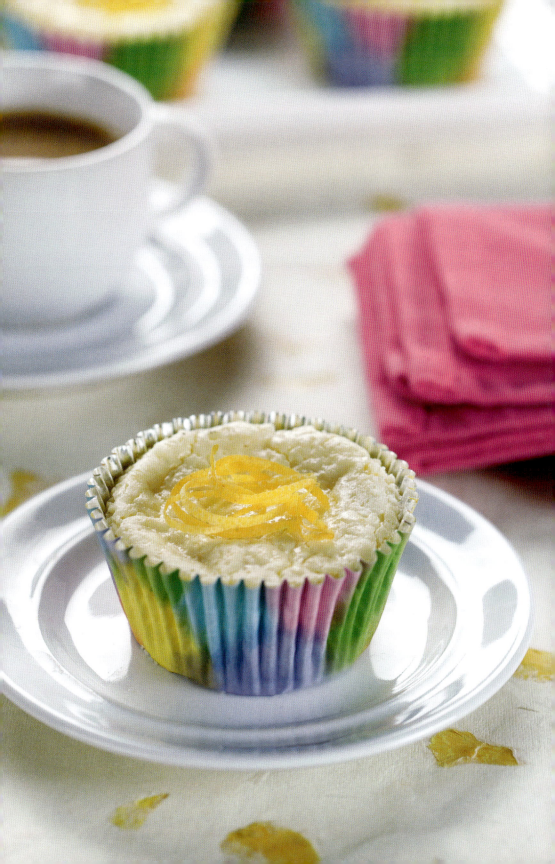

FIG BARS

Makes 12 servings (1 bar per serving)

FILLING

- ½ **cup dried figs**
- 6 **tablespoons hot water**
- 1 **tablespoon granulated sugar**

DOUGH

- ⅔ **cup all-purpose flour**
- ½ **cup quick oats**
- ¾ **teaspoon baking powder**
- ¼ **teaspoon salt**
- 2 **tablespoons oil**
- 3 **tablespoons fat-free (skim) milk**

ICING

- 1 **ounce reduced-fat cream cheese**
- ⅓ **cup powdered sugar**
- ½ **teaspoon vanilla**

1 Preheat oven to 400°F. Spray cookie sheet with nonstick cooking spray.

2 Combine figs, water and granulated sugar in food processor or blender; process until figs are finely chopped. Set aside.

3 Combine flour, oats, baking powder and salt in medium bowl. Add oil and just enough milk, 1 tablespoon at a time, until mixture forms a ball.

4 On lightly floured surface, roll dough into 12×9-inch rectangle. Place dough on prepared cookie sheet. Spread fig mixture in 2½-inch-wide strip lengthwise down center of rectangle. Make cuts almost to filling at ½-inch intervals on both 12-inch sides. Fold strips over filling, overlapping and crossing in center. Bake 15 to 18 minutes or until lightly browned.

5 Meanwhile, combine cream cheese, powdered sugar and vanilla in small bowl; mix well. Drizzle over bars. Cut into 12 pieces to serve.

Nutrition Information (per serving)

Calories 104, **Total Fat** 3g, **Saturated Fat** 1g, **Cholesterol** 1mg, **Sodium** 93mg, **Carbohydrates** 18g, **Dietary Fiber** 1g, **Protein** 2g

Dietary Exchanges: 1 Bread/Starch • ½ Fat

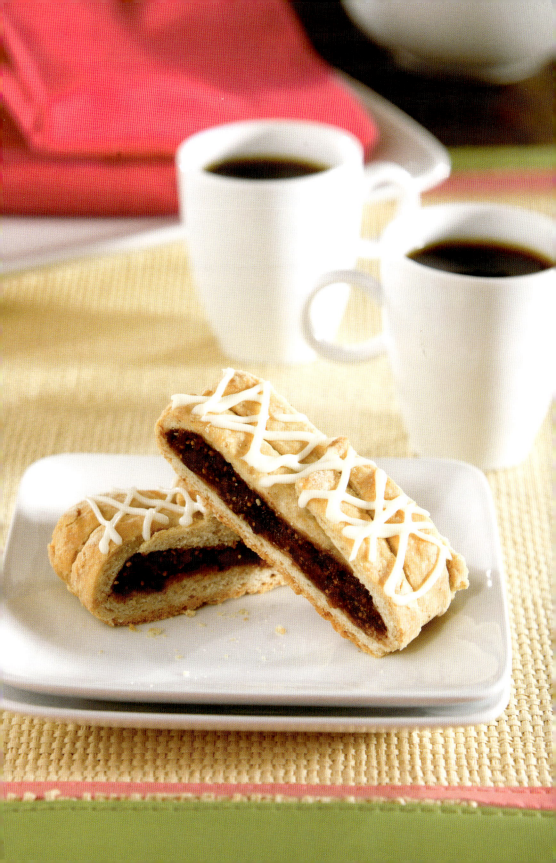

RUSTIC APPLE TART

Makes 8 servings

1 refrigerated pie crust (half of 14-ounce package)

4 medium Granny Smith apples, peeled, cored and thinly sliced (about 4 cups)

2 tablespoons packed brown sugar

¼ teaspoon ground cinnamon

1 egg white

3 tablespoons apricot fruit spread

1 Preheat oven to 375°F. Line baking sheet with parchment paper; spray with nonstick cooking spray.

2 Roll out pie crust on lightly floured surface to 12-inch circle. Place on prepared baking sheet.

3 Combine apples, brown sugar and cinnamon in large bowl; toss to coat evenly. Arrange apples in center of pie crust to within 1-inch of edge. Fold crust over apples. Brush with egg white.

4 Bake 25 minutes. Dot with fruit spread. Bake 5 to 10 minutes or until apples are crisp-tender and crust is golden brown. Let stand 5 minutes before cutting. Serve warm.

Nutrition Information (per serving)

Calories 160, **Total Fat** 6g, **Saturated Fat** 2g, **Cholesterol** 3mg, **Sodium** 137mg, **Carbohydrates** 26g, **Dietary Fiber** 1g, **Protein** 1g

Dietary Exchanges: 1 Bread/Starch • ½ Fruit • 1 Fat

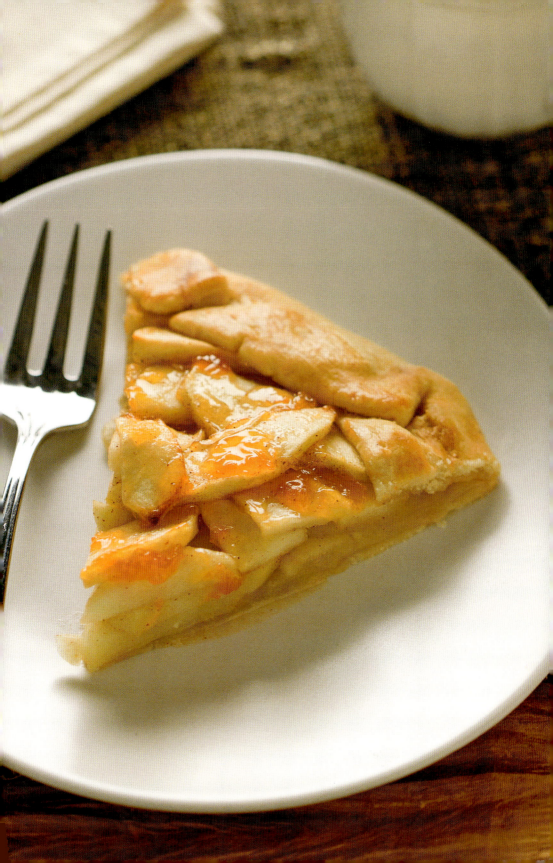

METRIC CONVERSION CHART

VOLUME MEASUREMENTS (dry)

1/8 teaspoon = 0.5 mL
1/4 teaspoon = 1 mL
1/2 teaspoon = 2 mL
3/4 teaspoon = 4 mL
1 teaspoon = 5 mL
1 tablespoon = 15 mL
2 tablespoons = 30 mL
1/4 cup = 60 mL
1/3 cup = 75 mL
1/2 cup = 125 mL
2/3 cup = 150 mL
3/4 cup = 175 mL
1 cup = 250 mL
2 cups = 1 pint = 500 mL
3 cups = 750 mL
4 cups = 1 quart = 1 L

VOLUME MEASUREMENTS (fluid)

1 fluid ounce (2 tablespoons) = 30 mL
4 fluid ounces (1/2 cup) = 125 mL
8 fluid ounces (1 cup) = 250 mL
12 fluid ounces (1 1/2 cups) = 375 mL
16 fluid ounces (2 cups) = 500 mL

WEIGHTS (mass)

1/2 ounce = 15 g
1 ounce = 30 g
3 ounces = 90 g
4 ounces = 120 g
8 ounces = 225 g
10 ounces = 285 g
12 ounces = 360 g
16 ounces = 1 pound = 450 g

DIMENSIONS

1/16 inch = 2 mm
1/8 inch = 3 mm
1/4 inch = 6 mm
1/2 inch = 1.5 cm
3/4 inch = 2 cm
1 inch = 2.5 cm

OVEN TEMPERATURES

250°F = 120°C
275°F = 140°C
300°F = 150°C
325°F = 160°C
350°F = 180°C
375°F = 190°C
400°F = 200°C
425°F = 220°C
450°F = 230°C

BAKING PAN SIZES

Utensil	Size in Inches/Quarts	Metric Volume	Size in Centimeters
Baking or Cake Pan (square or rectangular)	8×8×2	2 L	20×20×5
	9×9×2	2.5 L	23×23×5
	12×8×2	3 L	30×20×5
	13×9×2	3.5 L	33×23×5
Loaf Pan	8×4×3	1.5 L	20×10×7
	9×5×3	2 L	23×13×7
Round Layer Cake Pan	8×1½	1.2 L	20×4
	9×1½	1.5 L	23×4
Pie Plate	8×1¼	750 mL	20×3
	9×1¼	1 L	23×3
Baking Dish or Casserole	1 quart	1 L	—
	1½ quart	1.5 L	—
	2 quart	2 L	—